GRACIE'S STORY

Fighting to Survive Breast Cancer

Dear Coni
I lived to tell about it
and I'm talking!

Gracie
J.

GRACE A. WILSON-THOMPSON

This book is especially dedicated to ...

My three precious boys: Gregory, Tye, and Liam;
My beloved parents: Frank & Henny

and

My 'big' brother Franny.

And as a last minute dedication to Darlene,
who at the start of writing this book
was diagnosed with colon cancer.
The news you just never want to hear.

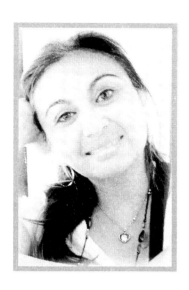

"Completely vulnerable and honest with myself and unapologetic when it comes to how I express myself in my medium. Some find me challenging when I am just being myself. Yet I end up touching and inspiring a lot of people. There are a lot of people I dearly love, admire, and respect. The biggest statement I could give to the world is to be strong being myself. And particularly at this time, more than ever before, when previously I most often put myself second, it is my priority and duty, and I owe it to myself to now only focus on me first! Speaking from my heart, there is no competition."

GRACIE

Acknowledgments

Special thanks to all my family, close friends, and colleagues for your support, thoughts, and prayers that the boys and I have received and continue to receive. While I have done pretty much everything on my own for the greatest part of my life and as a single mother of three, it was a humbling experience to have to surrender to all the help I was receiving. Looking back now, I know I could not have done any of what I have been through (treatments, the setback, etc.) without your unwavering help and support. No one fights alone! I am and always will be eternally grateful.

Heartfelt thanks to all the physicians—most particularly Dr. Le, Dr. Liu, Dr. Bajnrauh, Dr. Kato, and Dr. Shukla—nurses, and staff for the best care I've received.

Special thanks to contributing editor, Melissa Se

Contents

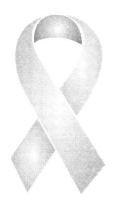

Introduction:

The Day Cancer Got Personal

I had been working in the trenches for various cancer, AIDS, cardiovascular disease, stroke awareness, and so on, when the unthinkable happened—one of the diseases I had fought to raise awareness for became more than just a cause. It was cancer, the big "C" word no one wants to mention out of fear that it will somehow step into their lives. But there I was, a single, 47-year-old mother of three with a heart for other people and a family halfway across the world starting my own reluctant cancer journey.

I am pleased to report that after a full year of battling the odds with Stage 3 breast cancer, I am a new woman. Now I have an amazing opportunity to share my experiences with you—the newly diagnosed man or woman that has to face a similar storm. And it is a storm—one of physical and emotional reactions, trials, adjustments, and facing challenges head on with all the support that you can get.

Through this journey I learned to continue laughing, which was such a big part of my recovery. Staying positive and rejoicing through the obstacles became my way of including my friends and family in the process. I kept a website so that one day I could let you know that everything will be all right.

The scariest part of cancer is the *unknown*. When you share your experience with others and do so with a happy heart, it lightens your own burden. This book is for the person currently battling with the despair of their diagnosis. It is for the family of the cancer patient that does not know what is going to happen or how they will get through it. I have drawn closer to my family and friends through this experience and have even picked up new friends along the way. The trick is to free your heart and focus on the things that encourage happiness, laughter, and love in your life so that you are equipped with enough armor to take on this deeply personal threat. The day cancer got personal, my life changed, but I continued to remain resolutely happy—and you can too. It is only a matter of perspective, hope, and choosing to walk down the right paths. Respect yourself enough to understand that a positive attitude is a healing one. This is the path you were meant to take. Will you follow me there?

She is clothed with *strength & dignity*, & she *laughs* without fear of the *future*.
-Proverbs 31:25

"Gracie, you are a warrior; there are no setbacks or losses. Only causes worth fighting for. Every unexpected turn is an opportunity to grow and discover another wonderful facet of yourself"
IG

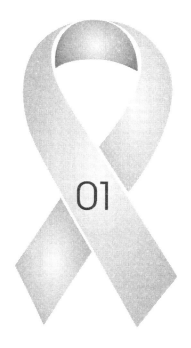

01

Changing Pace

*"You're going to go through tough times—that's life.
But I say, 'Nothing happens to you, it happens for
you.' See the positive in negative events."*
JOEL OSTEEN

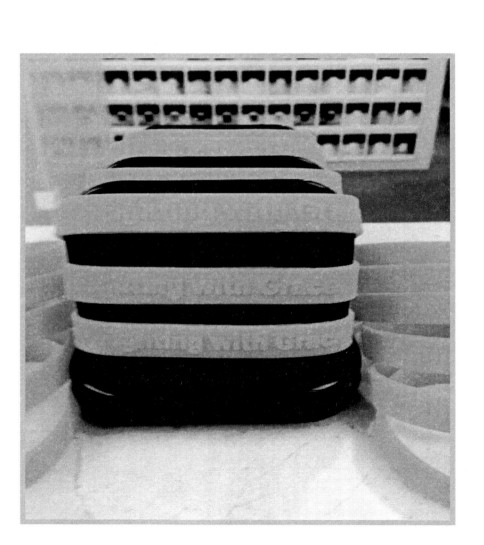

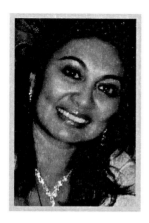

My name is Grace—most call me Gracie—and I have seen the real nature of cancer. Before my diagnosis, I was your average loving mom of three wonderful boys that I raised alone. After 16 years of marriage, and being together for nearly 20, I knew the time had come to start over somewhere new. At the time, there were only Gregory and Tye. It was a given that they come with me, and it was the best move I could have made for myself and the boys. The separation was nothing short of amicable and with respect. Deciding to pick up our lives and move from Florida to Arizona in 2006 was a hard decision to make. Any single mom will tell you that moving a child is tough—well, moving two across the country was no picnic! But I knew that we needed a fresh start in a place where we had never been before, where no one knew who we were.

A clean slate can be a very healing thing. So the three of us packed up our bags and made the necessary preparations to leave Florida. I had found a nice house on Craigslist that we could rent, and I arranged to have our paltry nine boxes of worldly possessions shipped to the Arizona house. It was going to be a whole new life for us, and we were very excited about it! At the time, I could never have imagined what my future had in store for me, but looking back, I am so glad that it led me here. Changing pace was something I needed after my marriage ended, and the boys were happy to strike out into the world and make their mark.

We arrived and moved into our new home in a quiet neighborhood in the Foothills, almost secluded right on the far south border of the big city. A family-friendly area with some of the best schools in the district nearby, it was a comfortable place to call home, and we settled in with little trouble. I began the "grand" search for work and was able to find a job in only a few short weeks, which was a definite blessing.

I am also a Buddhist, which means that I try to focus on doing things that make me feel good. This translates into doing and being good to other people who need a helping hand. There is no greater gift that you can give someone than the gift of support when they really need it, no matter how that manifests. To make others feel good about themselves, without judgment, is a life goal that I continue to pursue to this day. You would be amazed how much a single smile means to a cancer patient that has just had to sit through their fourth round of chemotherapy treatment. Smiles are so contagious, and I believe that it is our duty in this world to pass them around as much as possible. Misery only breeds more misery, and when the chips are down and your mind has sunk into despair, a friendly chat or a warm smile can restore the happiness that is supposed to be in someone's heart.

Throughout my journey, I was determined to be irrationally positive so that it would be as contagious as possible. Arizona was a great place to live until we hit another snag in the road—*the recession*. When the recession struck, a lot of people lost their jobs. I was one of them. In February 2008 I was officially without work, and no one was hiring. The next 18 months were some of the most humbling and difficult that I have ever experienced, but I got through them.

There is a helplessness that comes along with not being able to find a job that is similar to the despair that you feel when you are diagnosed with cancer. It was a heavy burden to bear with two sons who had a lot of needs that had to be taken into account. During my time as an unemployed person who was impacted by the recession,

I learned to put my pride aside and do what needed to be done. This meant accepting welfare and asking for help from a variety of different sources. Clothes, toiletries, utilities, and food-bank queues became our normal. I still remember the odd day that we did not have access to electricity or water. Those days reminded me that what most people consider "average" is actually truly remarkable.

Water does not need to be fetched from anywhere to be used. We just pay for it, and it comes out of our taps. Electricity is readily available for every modern convenience, but most people would be completely unable to live without it. On those cold, lean days, I reminded myself that this would not be my "forever" as long as I kept searching for work. I was a mother, and any fierce mom will tell you that when children are involved, there is no time for a pity party. Instead, we kick into high gear and do not divert from that until our children's needs are satisfied. And so I stood in food bank queues to collect the charity that so many people fail to recognize as a serious blessing. That charity got my family through some very harsh months, when food—the sustenance you need to speak, walk, and exist—was not something I could afford on my own.

Then to make this time more challenging is when I found myself expecting and had to dig deep within my mind, heart, and soul to make a choice. It then became a question I had to answer of what can I live with for the rest of my life? Ultimately, it came down to what we call the secret of happiness, which is no more a secret than our willingness to choose life! So in April of 2010 Gregory, Tye, and I joyfully welcomed our beautiful little son/brother, Liam. It is a decision I will never regret. He is my youngest and brings me additional joy and peace, makes my world complete, and makes all my battles worth fighting. I did not let the recession dash my hopes for our move to Arizona. It was a minor setback that I knew would one day come to an end. And it did!

One day in 2010, amidst the daily unemployment struggles, I finally landed a job—a good one with a large company—and that meant job security for the long term! Through hard work, my work ethic, integrity, dedication, and loyalty, I expect I will no longer have to look for employment, ideally, ever again! I have been with this company ever since, and I can honestly say that it was worth the wait. The friends and support structures that I have found there have seen me through the best and worst days of my cancer treatment. I would gladly pay those 18 months of living modestly to have discovered the great fortune that was waiting for me at my current employer. From that day on, I knew that things would be all right. Even when they become worse than you could ever imagine or expect, there is always light at the end of a tunnel. I insist on being the example to my boys so that they can see how courage, strength, patience, and endurance should be used to overcome life's most difficult challenges. These traits are needed most when the light has vanished and you are in for dark days. Choosing to be the only source of that light can make any experience better. That is the most fundamental truth I know.

Looking back on those leaner days on welfare, I am glad that they happened. They gave me the opportunity to teach my boys something valuable about life and the challenges that tend to arise. If I had chosen to internalize my failure to find a job, it would have destroyed me and made my situation worse. I would never have found my current job or the family that came with it. When life has stripped you of all you hold dear, a positive attitude will lift you out of that slump sooner than anything else. It is what landed me that fateful job, and it continues to be my greatest ally in the war against cancer. It is also a narrow path and one that few people can follow with conviction.

I am sure that the last thing on your mind is something positive if you have learned that your future is going to be littered with some very real challenges. But that is exactly why you need that positive outlook. So much of the challenge with cancer is learning about your own frailty and how much of the Journey you will need to walk alone. While you may be surrounded by family and friends, ultimately, the cancer belongs to you. Because of this, it stirs up feelings of mortality, despair, hopelessness, and panic—and these just love to emerge at inconvenient times. Having a positive attitude when you have cancer is a constant struggle. But believe me when I say that it is one that will draw the light closer when it seems so far off.

When everything around you has gone dark, *you* can be the source of your own light. Shine it on others, and do not obsess about the little things that are making your life harder. You have to thrive to survive. Best case scenario, you recover completely from cancer and get to write a book one day yourself. Worst case scenario, your final life Journey is undertaken with courage, grace, and laughter, and you do not spend your remaining days in despair. It sounds like a good deal to me however you look at it—which is where I placed my faith.

Many people know I am passionate about raising awareness for people who are dealing with difficult illnesses. AIDS, cancer, stroke, and cardiovascular disease were the main issues on the agenda. I would be the one encouraging people to participate in the various events with me and make donations. In my position as an Executive Assistant, I know many people and know of a lot of resources, and it is easy for me to bring people together and build teams to participate in the various events and donation efforts.

Sometimes I feel like my Journey took me to that position on purpose. When I was diagnosed with cancer, I was completely alone in Arizona—all of my family members, childhood friends, and closest friends were somewhere far away, either abroad or out of state. This meant that Gregory, my eldest son, had to face some challenges of his own. And what a rock he was and continues to be for our little family! At 16 years old, he embraced the reality of the situation and cared for his younger brothers, Tye and Liam. When I could no longer smile through the treatment, he was always there to push the cloud aside and let the light back in. I am proud to say that the lessons he learned during our time without money and support nearby served him well when I was diagnosed with cancer.

An old soul, Gregory has seen me knocked down in life, but all three, including Tye and Liam, always see me get back up. It greatly minimized their worries and fears! I am glad to have passed on this trait, and it has been a blessing to our family during these long, hard days. That is why I strongly advise anyone dealing with the realities of cancer to find that rock—someone super close to you that will lift you out of the emotional quagmire so that you can continue to fight even when you feel like you have to stop.

Laughing through the experience has brought me a lot of comfort as well. With something as serious as cancer, people forget that laughter is actual medicine. Keeping yourself happy is a way to stay strong and face the rough seas. This is a decision that you need to make for the good of your family and for your own recovery. It is not a decision that can be thrust on you, because as I mentioned earlier, cancer has a way of dragging you down. If you are already down, things will only become harder, and soon you will face a wall of the impossible instead of believing in your positive outcome.

At the same time, I want to express my eternal gratitude for the people in my life who have kept the light shining on me. My father Frank—a proud and true Asian cultured disciplinary man, whom I highly respect and love dearly and with all of my heart. My utmost priority in life has been and always will be to make him proud—even when I know he already is! My mother Henny, whom I love and respect equally as much, a worrywart who continuously needed my strength and optimism to realize that all things have an end. "All will be well, Mama!" I always tell her. My brother Franny, who is a man of few words but who has kept me in his prayers, day in, day out. For the many close friends who flocked to help me when they discovered the challenges that I would have to face—a deeper, more sincere thank you I could never offer you!

Your family and close friends act as shields between you and your diagnosis. You cannot hope to conquer cancer alone, because it is a very destructive thing. Luckily, I was able to motivate my friends and family on my good days, who in turn could motivate me on my bad ones. While this Journey has been one I will never forget, the outpouring of love and support that I have felt is irreplaceable. No one fights alone!

Despite cancer being something that will always be a part of my life story, it will never define me. Instead, the experiences that I have gleaned from the days in chemotherapy, during the surgeries, and after radiation treatments will become a part of me. All the support, love, and sacrifice that I was shown have already healed me. And now that I am doing okay, I am free to begin my Journey to help you. Because when you help someone else with cancer, it makes yours seem insignificant. When you help someone see the bright side of a dark experience, it comes back to you tenfold. I believe that, and I am standing here stronger because of it.

As you read this story, I urge you to begin one of your own. Do not see your cancer experience as a negative thing but as an opportunity to explore the strongest aspects of what makes you who you are, and then share it with others. Cancer is horrible, and it may very well be the worst thing that ever happens to you. But it does not have to steal away your joy. It should put that joy on a stage and let it light the way forward.

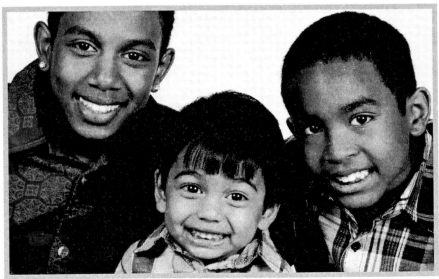

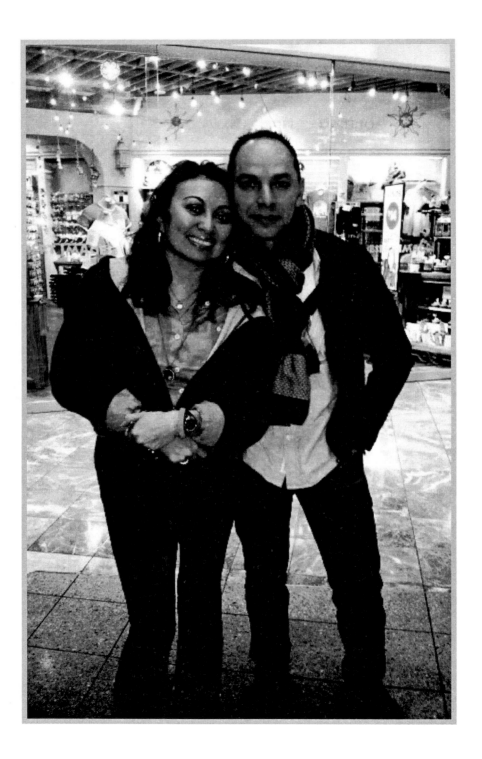

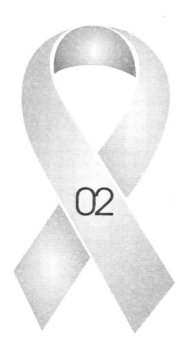

02

My Formal Diagnosis

*"Cancer is so limited...it cannot cripple love, it
cannot shatter hope, it cannot corrode faith, it
cannot destroy peace, it cannot kill friendship, it
cannot suppress memories, it cannot silence courage,
it cannot invade the soul, it cannot steal eternal life,
it cannot conquer the spirit."*
AUTHOR UNKNOWN

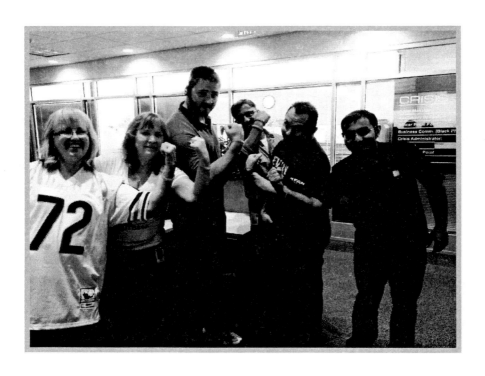

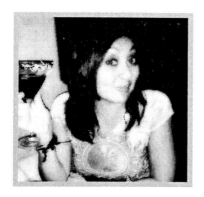

It was a normal day back in April 2013 when I scheduled a routine mammogram for myself. It is never a pleasant screening test, but like many other things in life, it is necessary to make sure that your health is still on track. During the mammogram, your breast is placed between two plates and is squeezed in the machine. The X-ray is then taken when the breast tissue is thin enough, and in 20 minutes, it is all over. It is a silly test really, when nothing appeared to be out of the ordinary. So I did not worry. Some six months later, I realized something was wrong on discovery of a hard lump and immediately contacted Dr. Le, my primary care physician, the very next morning, who ordered a mammogram and ultrasound stat. Within that same day, within just a few hours really, I received that dreadful call from him that he was very sorry and that the lump was very likely cancerous. He referred me that same week to Dr. Liu, a breast cancer specialist, who ordered two more mammograms, two ultrasounds, an MRI, and three biopsies in tow—the diagnosis was official: *I had breast cancer.*

And it was not just any breast cancer, but Stage 3 breast cancer. The tumor discovered was not 2 ½ centimeters as initially measured but 5½ centimeters—making it a much later stage of cancer. I remember hearing the diagnosis from the doctor for the first time. Like many patients, after hearing "cancer," my mind went blank, and I barely have any memories of what the doctor said afterwards. It did not sink in until several days later, but I was determined not to let this obstacle defeat me.

One of the first things I did was call my father. It had always been a priority in my life to make him proud, and we had a long conversation about it on the phone. "Gracie, no pity! You are born a warrior, and you are going to fight! Do whatever it is you need to do to get through this. You have a responsibility! Think of your children, and show them what courage, strength, patience, and endurance mean!"

The news slowly tore through my family like a tsunami. The boys took the diagnosis hard, but I spent a lot of time making sure that they knew nothing was going to happen to me. I would fight with every ounce of strength I had. "Mama was not going anywhere!" I pondered over my Stage 3 diagnosis and became resolute to beat it. Stage 3 is when the cancer has spread beyond the immediate region of the tumor and could be invading nearby lymph nodes and muscles— but no other organs yet.

As the days rolled by, there were questions from every corner, and these only bred more questions. I made the decision to keep an online journal of my journey fighting cancer so that my family and friends could all be updated about it at once. My parents, brother, and other important people in my life could keep "abreast" of what was happening with me there on a practically day-to-day basis. This would help limit the worry that my parents and brother had, and because they could not travel, it became a great way to communicate with them, even during the hardest parts of the recovery period. Everyone was concerned that with no real family in Arizona (or anywhere in the U.S. for that matter), I would not have enough support and would not make it through my recovery alone. Fortunately, fate had brought me to an extraordinary team of people that I worked with, and they essentially became my family during this process. During the times when I was too weak to write in the journal, my friend Linda would write the updates on the journal. And so my personal community of friends and family sprang up with my website, Graciesfight.com.

On my very first page on this website, I welcome everyone and thank them for joining me in my battle against breast cancer. From the first page I wrote, "I WILL live to tell you all about it!" and I have. So think of this book as a way that I can communicate with my family in greater detail while sharing my Journey with a greater audience of people—people like you, who have been impacted by cancer and do not know how to deal with it. My hope is that my fight will inspire you to stage one of your own. This is how we survive and conquer!

After my formal diagnosis, I went through the seven stages of grief, like everyone is forced to when faced with a life-threatening illness. Launching the website was a big part of my acceptance stage, and I knew it was the right thing to do to keep myself going. I have always been the kind of person who needs to reach out and help others. I have never been great at being helped, so the emotions of the experience were overwhelming at times.

I want to impress upon you how important it is for you to reach the "acceptance and hope" stage quickly. The other stages are painful, and while it has to be experienced to truly understand, having cancer is really mind over matter. There is no point making it worse for yourself by harping on your tumors every five minutes and realizing once again that they are trying to kill you. I spent a long time feeling betrayed by my body, like it had turned against me and I no longer had control over what was happening in my life. But—and believe me when I say this—cancer is not about control.

Once you are diagnosed, you know you are not well, regardless of how you feel. You may have been ill, or you may not feel ill at all. Whatever the case, you will have to go through some unsavory treatments to save your life. Illness is in your future. That does not mean you have to invite it into your life right away however. Hold onto the moments of calm, pain-free living while you can. It will make the other moments better when they happen. Otherwise you will spend the entire length of time, perhaps several years, battling with your cancer in a perpetual state of panic and misery. I am sure I do not have to tell you how this impacts your survival chances. Happier people survive cancer more easily because they are able to keep that panic away and see things more clearly. I am not saying that you cannot do it in despair, but it is definitely a more harrowing experience. Once I knew that cancer was in me, I needed to focus on getting it out.

Everyone has their own cancer diagnosis story. I want to encourage you to use yours to connect with other cancer patients as you meet them along your Journey. They are normal people who were hit with the shocking moment themselves, and it will help them to share that moment with someone who understands it. No routine mammogram ever starts out as a cancer mammogram. No emergency room visit, doctor's appointment, or standard screening ever begins as a cancer discovery session.

We all share the same fear about it, and sharing that fear lightens the emotional load. I know a lot of good people who have made it through their treatment because they found friends going through the same thing. It helps to have a support group, inside and outside of the disease. That way you get to focus on what matters without always feeling like the cancer is taking over your life (which it does).

Being diagnosed with cancer can cause a lot of different emotions to rise up in you. You may be afraid that your family will suffer without you or fearful that you did not take advantage of life while you had it. Whatever your feelings, acknowledge them and write them down. You do not have to talk about them all the time, but sharing them this way makes them real, and you can close the "book" on them so to speak. This leaves room for you to continue choosing to feel positive about your diagnosis once you reach that point. And you will. With any cancer diagnosis, there are only two routes you can take—*life or death*.

If you plan on choosing life, you may as well choose it with a heart full of joy. Living like you are going to die and then surviving only robs you of your chance to make your life better during those tough days. Above all, you will face this question many times—continue… or game over?—like one of my son's computer games. Always know that your default is continue. Remind yourself, suck it up, and consciously do your best to keep going.

I accepted my cancer diagnosis, although it was terrifying and crippling to do it. I could often feel myself wanting to panic about my sons and myself, but I refused to do that. The universe also sent me some real support, the lights that shone through those dark times and kept me going. There was Eddy, a long-standing childhood friend who flew to the U.S. to help me with no fantastical notions about an American vacation. He came at the exact time I needed someone to look after my boys at home after being unexpectedly and with rush admitted to the hospital with a Staph infection that left me down and out for nearly a week. Though I had not seen him in over 30 years, he was a blessing that I needed.

Then I had support from my boss Paul and all of his managers and staff, even beyond our department within the company. So many became near and dear friends after I was diagnosed. Many of them became more than just friends; we truly bonded as a family: Judi as the mother-figure, Linda as my father-figure, Kathleen as my sister-figure, and Jim G. as the older brother-figure to name some of the closest ones. It is impossible to name all my "brothers and sisters" I have gained along the way, and they all equally contributed to being the family I now have in all of them! But with Judi and Linda, as the "parents" they became to me, they sure kept me "walking on my toes" when I did not reveal a struggle and/or was stubborn doing something I was not supposed to do. And they quickly put me in my place when needed with their looks and tones of voice, just like my true parents would have if they were there. Though some have never had to deal directly with cancer before (no friends or family), they took turns going with me to every doctor's appointment. They all became my impromptu caregivers after surgery. The very first week

I spent at Linda's home, and she helped me take my medications, fed me, bathed me—everything I could ever have asked for. Her selflessness and care is something I am privileged to have in my life—everyone for that matter. Support is something every cancer patient needs, even if they do not want it. Without the people I have mentioned—and many more—I am sure my Journey would have been different. Judi constantly came over to look after me and the boys, and Kathleen was like the big sister I never had. My colleagues became my family, and to all of you, I express my deepest gratitude. Paul, Judi, Linda & Julio, Kathleen, Jim & Cissy, Jessica, Carla & Nate, Charlie & Darlene, Miki & Peggy, Julie, Mike V. Steven R., Zach & Jie, Llew, Randy, Kimberley, Erik, Justin, Dean, Rosemary, Dewayne, Keith, Todd, Eric, Karen, Darlene, Teena, Cheryl and Dennis "DJ"—all of you are so dear to me. There are so many of you that it is impossible for me to mention you all, but please know I did not and never will forget each and every one of you and what you have done for me and the boys! That being said, if you do not have a strong support base, you need to get one.

I was and am so blessed. I even had Mary, who sent me handwritten postcards with photographs that she made for me *every* single day—there were times when I received three on the same day! And then there was Judith, who came into town on business, took time out to come over to my home, and cooked for me and the boys. All of this helped fuel my stubbornly positive spirit, something you must have for the coming battle ahead. People cannot be sidelined or alienated during this Journey—though you will have plenty of reason to do it. Just do not!

I want to urge you not to discount the value of a single smile as you move through your treatment. Recovery will be rough, but it can also be fun. Good memories of bringing people closer, sharing yourself, being cared for, and spreading positive messages of hope are what could be in your future if you only dare to reach for them.

Now that I am on the other side of the storm, I can tell you—smiling through it was valuable. Being upset, panicked, and in a perpetual state of confusion and despair is not good for you. Your mindset matters during your recovery. While you did not ask to develop cancer, there are millions of other people that are going through it as well. You can either be a beacon of light to make their days easier or you can be the opposite and sink into an isolated despair. I remember cracking jokes at the most wonderful things. Once I had lost all of my hair, all that I could do was make bald jokes! Trying on wigs with Judi was such an epic event, and we laughed so much to the point that our stomachs and cheek muscles hurt. It lightened the mood and kept me in good spirits. Ultimately, that is your target emotional state.

If you can speak to the people in your life and communicate this to them while attempting to live as a positive human being with cancer, you can crush it. When you look to your left and see a person in tears or to your right to see another trying hard not to deal with what they are going through—I challenge you. Share yourself, and be positive. It will help you climb over the steepest hills, and in the end, you will all make it to the other side unscathed.

Now I am going to tell you what happened once I was diagnosed—the storm of options, information, and confusion that descended on me and how I dealt with it. For the next several chapters, I will recount my days and what I went through. I only hope that in this sharing, you find peace, calm, and the strength you need to face it yourself. Because you are strong—you just do not know it yet—and you will be surprised how much you can deal with when it is staring you straight in the face.

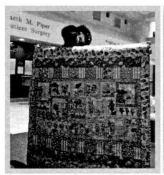
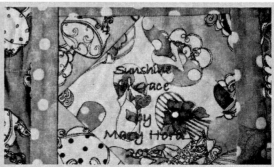

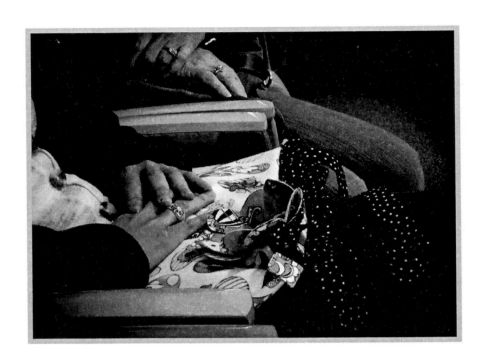

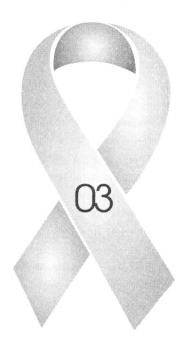

03

Make Mine a Double

*"You gain strength, courage, and confidence
by every experience in which you really stop
to look fear in the face. You must do the thing
which you think you cannot do."*
ELEANOR ROOSEVELT

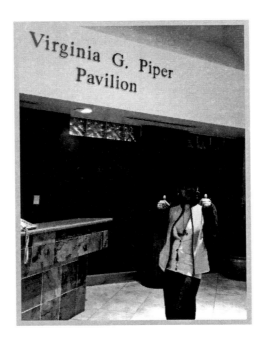

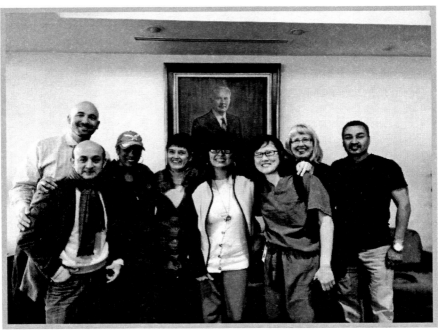

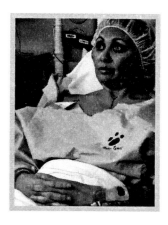

I was thrown into the deep end after my diagnosis. Before I had time to think, the doctor had scheduled me in for a double mastectomy, which would be followed by reconstructive surgery. I had to have both of my breasts removed, and I was quite attached to them after so many years! It was a lot to process, but as I have said before—cancer does not care about your control issues. Once it has reached a certain stage, you have to act fast.

On January 1, 2014, I wrote my first surgical entry on my online website. I reported that I was scheduled for surgery the next day at 11:00 a.m. The double mastectomy would take six hours to perform and was not going to be a walk in the park. This was my first big treatment after my diagnosis, and to be honest, I was not prepared for it. You may find yourself being ill prepared for a lot of cancer-related treatments, but that is normal. Stage 3 cancer does not wait to be treated; it is just treated or it kills you. So on the second day of 2014, I was met by some of my closest friends at the Scottsdale Virginia G. Piper Surgery Center. Quite an entourage and doctors and staff were surprised by it. Never before had they seen anything like this. They came from all different parts of the valley at such an early hour just to show their support! I was admitted to the hospital and underwent my double mastectomy.

When it was all over, Linda reported that I was resting in the recovery room at 6:15 p.m. Dr. Liu, the breast cancer specialist, had come in earlier that day to tell me there were no problems with the surgery. They had removed four lymph nodes, and the test came back negative for cancer. Everyone had been praying for me, and although I was in the hospital about to face the new day, I had all the support I needed. After the double mastectomy and reconstructive surgery, the plastic surgeon, Dr. Bajnrauh, told me that all had "gone well." However, the plan was to place implants, but a second tumor was discovered that had already traveled through the muscle, and Dr. Bajnrauh was not comfortable leaving it at that and had placed expanders instead. It is quite a shock when you hear that. During the ordeal, I resolutely expressed a positive attitude. By 10:30 that evening I was chatting to several friends who had stopped by the hospital. They told me that I would be released on Friday afternoon. The surgery took a lot out of me, but my emotional state was strong and compensated for my weakened physical state. I was on the mend!

When I was finally able to go home (well, Linda's home, that is, for the first couple of days), I was still in no shape to post on my website, so Linda did it for me. The night before I had a private hospital room all to myself and was enthusiastically speaking to people. Before I was released, Dr. Liu visited me and said that I was doing better than 80–90% of her patients! Clearly the positive attitude was an asset. I had to walk around for a bit and eat breakfast, and then I took a nap. Later that day I prepped for home! The drive home was worse than the surgery—every little bump felt like a massive boulder. The pain was worst at those moments.

Linda published widespread reports of "sleeping" activity because my pain medication had knocked me out. This was a really good thing because I was totally exhausted from the entire experience and needed some quality rest. Sleeping in a hospital is like pretend rest, with the real recovery occurring when you get home. I do not think anyone enjoys being in a hospital away from what they love and know. The best thing is to take the rest seriously, even if you feel like you do not want too. Rest! You have just been through something very traumatic, even if you were not awake to experience it. The Benadryl they put me on is a type of antihistamine, and it put me straight to sleep. Plus, it helped get rid of an itchy feeling I had post-surgery. The pain was there, but it was manageable.

I spent my day in a recliner, wrapped Eskimo-style in a warm quilt. I made sure that I ate because the doctors told me it would help my body tolerate the medication better. I was given a list of instructions to perform to keep myself moving and my lungs in good shape. I walked just a little and received the most beautiful flowers from friends. The constant stream of support from my website was an overwhelming comfort. I knew that I was not alone and that I would be well looked after. To me, that was more than enough.

By the time January 4 rolled around, I was feeling a lot better. The evening before had been comfortable and restful, and the pain medication was doing a fair job of controlling the pain that reared up every now and then. I found that I had renewed strength that morning and that sitting hurt a lot less than before. This was evidence that my body was healing, and I was glad. Plus, the irritating itching had gone away, which was a blessing. I focused on moving a little more and getting a lot more sleep. Sleep is very healing after a massive surgery; I highly recommend that you take it seriously despite what your brain might want.

With Linda's help, I continued to make sure that I was well fed, and I was fortunate to not experience any nausea that patients commonly have from the medication. I also performed my breathing exercises like a pro and got a surprise package from my friends over at work. They custom ordered and distributed nearly 250 pink "Fighting with Grace" rubber wristbands, which are undoubtedly the coolest things I have ever owned. I had enough strength to complain heartily about the hospital socks I was given, so my sense of humor was still firmly intact. The good news is that surgery does not impact your cheerful disposition.

The day after that I felt even better—growing in strength. I went for quite some time without that pain medication, which was also excellent. I went for another morning walk, and the last few itchy patches cleared up. These days were solely focused on healing, which meant that I had to stick to the basics—eating, doctor exercising (which is like exercising only prescribed by a doctor, and it is much harder than normal), sleeping, and chatting with a few visitors. By that evening I was comfortable enough to relax. I enjoyed being fussed over by Jessica and Judi and, of course, Linda—who made sure that I was never without anything. Following these healing protocols was tough because tiredness becomes something that hits you in your bones. But I managed it, and you will too. Just remember to rise in the morning with a smile, and seize every opportunity to share it with someone else.

By January 6 the surgery was almost fully behind me—what a difference a single day can make to your body! I was up that morning, took a nice long shower, and had something of a photo-shoot to share with my friends and family online—a 10-second video Linda's husband Julio made laughing, a little dance and singing: "I'm walking! I'm walking!" I felt renewed energy and was able to do more, plus I took far less pain medication, which addles your brain. I scheduled my post-operative visit with Dr. Bajnrauh and had a great day. I say "great" because I was awake to see most of it. Even I was surprised at how good I felt.

When the following day came around, I was thrilled at how strong I felt. I immediately took to the website to check it out after performing my rituals—eating, walking, doctor exercising, and chatting. My boys would finally be coming home from their winter break in Florida the next day, so I was in good spirits. That night I slept extremely well knowing that I had a doctor's appointment the next day and would get to see the boys.

The morning came, and off I went to see Dr. Bajnrauh, my plastic surgeon. He examined me and said that I was looking great! The incisions were healing well, and he removed the time release pain medication ball. We rescheduled to see each other every five weeks, and soon I was back in my own home waiting for the boys. Linda and her husband Julio had given me some tasty new food items to try, but I enjoyed unpacking and settling back in. I ran a few important errands (hey, life does not stop!) and then picked up Lyani, my awesome and oh so sweet dog, and brought her home. I barely needed any pain medication at all. On Friday I was scheduled to see Dr. Liu again to get my new pathology results. Then the boys arrived! I went to sleep very late because I was so excited to see them. Even though we were all tired, me from my surgery and them from the flight home, we stayed up together for a long time. I managed to sleep from midnight to 5:30 a.m. and then helped the boys get ready for school. The thing about cancer is that it tends to invade your normal life, which does not stop. You have to keep going with the dailies, which can be a struggle in the beginning.

Once the boys left for school on the bus, I went back to sleep. I woke for lunch and felt good. The only pain I felt was like the pain you feel the morning after a tough session at the gym—tight muscles and an achy feeling. I only took one to two Vicodin at night to help me sleep and one to two Tylenol in the morning. I was prescribed an antibiotic, which I was still taking. I stopped taking the Valium as soon as I could, very shortly after the surgery. I worked hard at being disciplined enough to not do anything I was not supposed to do. It was incredibly hard, but I had to heal correctly for my family.

The double mastectomy was my own choice. Typically, Dr. Liu does not recommend a double mastectomy very quickly, but she commended me on my choice—"That was a great call there, Gracie!"—as pathology test results did show atypical cells in the left breast that could have potentially become cancerous later on. All I was thinking when making the choice is that I never wanted to find myself in this predicament again. I would do whatever needed to be done to never have to worry if or when cancer would appear in the other breast. As previously mentioned, during surgery, another cancerous tumor was discovered, which she retracted. It was an unusual case, and she had to remove additional tissue, skin, and muscle—scary stuff! Dr. Liu removed four lymph nodes from the right breast, but all of them were negative for cancer.

Dr. Liu planned on presenting my case at the next Board of Cancer Specialists (oncologists, radiologists, surgeons, etc.) meeting because it was so unusual. We spoke about chemotherapy and radiation treatments and more tests. I left with the hope that I would not have to go through that, but I was prepared for anything. The next day was freezing cold. The shivering hurt, especially in my right breast—which made chatting to visitors harder than I would have liked. A slight throbbing pain set in, and I learned a lesson. Do not go outside in the cold after major surgery. So as the week wore on, I kept myself warm so that I did not shiver and cause havoc in my wounds. I felt no pain, which was awesome, so I did not even have to take any Tylenol. I did become frustrated that I had limited mobility though. I am usually a busy person, and I wanted to do so much more than I could. This, I believe, was the biggest struggle for me at the time: restraint. The boys were at school, and between visitors, I had to work hard to do nothing, or I would risk injuring myself.

On January 14 I woke to a total lack of energy, the consequence of doing too much the day before (even though I barely did anything!). I just could not sleep that evening, so I slept for most of the day after dropping the boys at school. I went through the motions of my doctor-approved schedule and sank back into dreamland.

The next day I met with Dr. Bajnrauh, my plastic surgeon, who told me I was looking wonderful. He removed the right drain but left the other one in. These drains remove the fluid, and if they come out early, they can cause infection, which would invoke an entirely new reconstructive process. The process of expanding the expanders placed on both sides had started, and it did not hurt. Every couple of weeks they would be expanded, with the left breast going at half the pace of the right.

The next two days were great, with the hardest part being the wait for the Board of Specialists panel to consult on my case. I felt really upbeat and energetic and had no pain at all. I did not take Ibuprofen for muscle aches at all. I continued with my regular doctor-prescribed walks and ate and drank to heal myself. The anxiety was creeping in about the radiation and chemotherapy treatments—I was dreading the determination.

Finally, I had one good, full day. I took the boys out for some well-deserved dim sum, a tradition that we tried to keep in our house because of our Chinese roots. It felt really good to be out of the house doing something normal with my family. I walked steadily but did not overdo it. You will find that keeping things slow and measured is so important to recovery. The rest of the day passed in a relaxing haze. I had no pain and was on no medication, and only a small tube reminded me of my surgery. It would fill up often, so I doubted that the doc would take it out at my next appointment. I smiled a lot and continued to be upbeat. That first normal day was so rejuvenating for me. And when you experience it, you will feel the same. There is nothing better than getting back to normal when you have had "abnormal" for so long.

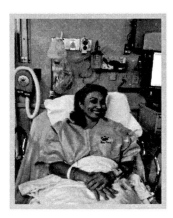
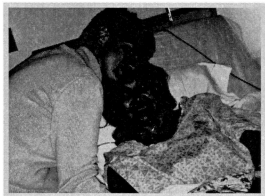

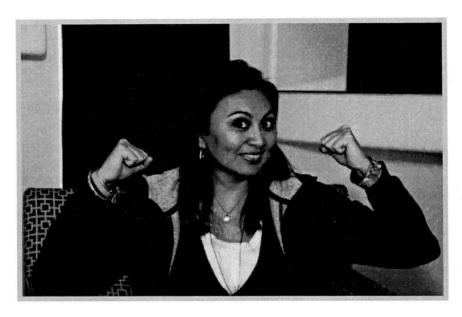

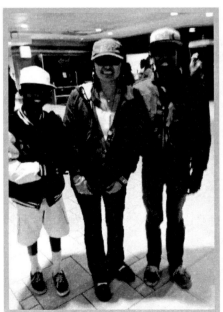

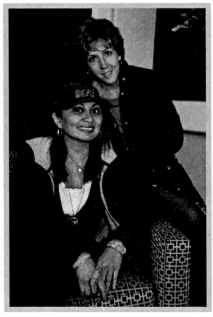

04

On the Road to Recovery

"Cancer is a journey, but you walk the road alone. There are many places to stop along the way and get nourishment—you just have to be willing to take it."
EMILY HOLLENBERG

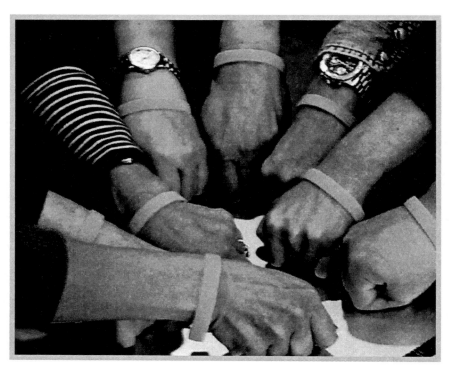

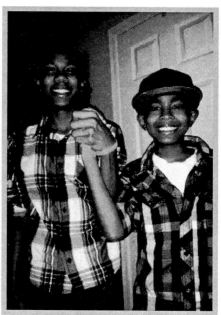

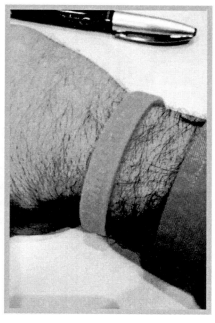

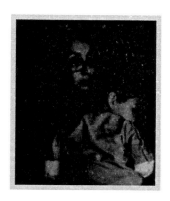

I saw Dr. Bajnrauh, my plastic surgeon. He said that all was coming along well. It was January 22, and I had been recovering and healing as I should be, which is always a positive sign! But he could not remove my drain on the left hand side because there was still a lot of fluid being produced there. I was told that it was normal to experience some delays with the drain removal, and when the fluid decreased, it would be removed. Dr. Bajnrauh took the time to explain the process of expanding my left side to me, and he continued to expand my right side. Because of the delay, the plan was to take it slow with the right to give the left hand side a chance to catch up.

During the week I often had tightness in my chest, but the process was simple, so it was not painful. The good news was that Dr. Bajnrauh was on the board that would decide whether or not I had to go for radiation treatment. While I was at the appointment, he explained to me what the board had discussed. They had met the night before and had decided that I needed both chemotherapy and radiation treatments. The chemotherapy was needed because the one tumor was embedded in the muscle tissue and there were cancer cells along the side of my breast there.

Radiation would be required to ensure that all cancer cells were killed. The board still needed to determine whether I would receive radiation on my entire chest area or more specific treatment. Dr.

Liu would let me know about the type of treatment that would be conducted.

The news was not a shock; I had a feeling deep in my gut that I would have to go for both chemotherapy and radiation treatment. A friend of mine told me that I took the news well, but as a strategic thinker, I knew that more treatment would be necessary. As long as I retained a healthy, positive attitude about it, there was nothing that could stop me from fully recovering from cancer. Dr. Bajnrauh would continue the reconstruction until the treatment was underway; then it would have to wait until all of the cancer was gone.

That night, I felt very tired, and I had a slight fever. By the morning, I was in the throes of chills and fever. My chest hurt from the expansion pain the day before, and I was completely out of commission. The following day was not much better. My fever subsided some, but I still felt sluggish. Sleep was difficult with the stretching expansion pain. I decided to stay in bed and get some rest and to drink lots of fluids. The following day, I decided to cruise around with Eddy to show him Apache Junction, visited the Lost Dutchman Mine ghost town, and took a walk down Mill Avenue. I paid for that exertion big time!

I was a total wipe out later after fully realizing that I would have to undergo chemotherapy and radiation. It dawns on you suddenly, even if you were expecting it. I decided to see Dr. Liu as soon as possible to get the ball rolling. The only problem was that the fluids from my left drain were increasing and were now sandy in color— not good. I took Tylenol to prevent fever, but the pain told me that something was wrong. Ibuprofen was not enough, and I had to take Vicodin to get around. I did not feel well, so I called Dr. Bajnrauh and told him as much.

Eddy, a longtime childhood friend whom I had not seen in over 30 years, came down from Holland to help me. He stayed in my home full time and made an incredible difference during this tough time. The following day the fluid became clear again, and I took it easy, scheduling both doctors' appointments for the same day.

The first appointment was with Dr. Liu, who confirmed that chemotherapy and radiation were necessary. I would have to do chemotherapy sessions for four months, and she would work on my radiation plan. Dr. Kato, the oncologist, would walk me through the chemotherapy plan the following week. My second appointment of the day was with Dr. Bajnrauh, and it turned out I had a major infection. I was instantly admitted to the hospital next door and put on antibiotics and pain medication.

The expansion was reduced to give me some relief. The infection in my left breast was severe, so Dr. Bajnrauh told me that he would decide soon whether surgery would be required to remove the expander from the infected area. I had some lovely visitors that day and received some wonderful flowers that lifted my spirits.

Suddenly, the following day, I was scheduled for surgery again. The night before my doctors had decided to remove the expander to get rid of the infection. I was put on stronger pain medication and slept until surgery, logging into pre-op at 1:00 p.m. Dr. Bajnrauh had a previously scheduled engagement out of state, so he handed his care over to his partner, Dr. Andres. Dr. Andres told me that he would replace the expander and install two drains instead of the normal one drain. The tissue would be examined for infection at the same time. The surgery went as well as can be expected, and Dr. Andres discovered a nasty Staph infection in my tissue that needed to be treated with antibiotics until February 14.

I slept through the night, exhausted from surgery and the pain medications. The following morning I had breakfast and returned to dreamland. My fever spiked to 103°F, and the doctors did what they could to treat me. They used ice packs to keep my temperature low, so I shivered relentlessly and had a giant headache. When I woke up from the deliria the next day, it was rough. My fever fluctuated between 100°F and 103°F. The headache would not go away—this was one stubborn infection!

My visitors kept me in good spirits while I worked to beat the infection, which tests showed was not in my blood. By February second I was finally feeling a bit better. My pain was less, but my iron levels were low from surgery, so I was given vitamins, potassium, and iron. Full of vitamins, I ate dinner and went to sleep. Eddy looked after the boys, which was such a blessing. The following day I did feel a little better—recovery comes in inches, not miles. I was more alert and could walk faster when awake.

Note: From the time that I was admitted to the hospital up until from this point forward when I was feeling better, I have absolutely no recollection of four days out of that one week's stay in the hospital! Linda wrote the updates on my website while I was "down and out."

Once I felt better, all I wanted to do was go home. They continued me on the vitamins, and the infection improved as well. The entire time I was dealing with the Staph infection I was lucky to have my friends and Eddy, who looked after my boys and me. Cancer can cause all kinds of complications, so you have to be on your toes for emergency hospital visits, especially if you have not been feeling well. Never ignore it! I ignored it for three days and paid for it by being admitted to the hospital and undergoing yet another surgery to have this serious infection removed and the replacement of an expander.

February 3 was a good day. The best medicine in the world came to visit me in the form of Eddy, Gregory, and Tye. It was a surprise visit, and it cheered me right up. After that they went out for Italian food to unwind, while I stayed in hospital. Eddy was so good with the boys, and it was exactly what I needed at the time. I even took a shower, I was in such good spirits. The bandages from surgery came off, and everything looked good. My red blood cell count needed to increase, so the medication was helping with that. I was so ready to go home, but I had to wait for the all clear.

The next day Dr. Bajnrauh came to visit, and he reduced my medication intake so that I could be more alert. My vitals were good, and the vitamins had made a difference. The more active I could be, the better, and I was told that I would be released soon. My boys and Eddy came for dinner that evening, and it was good to laugh with them again.

By February 5 I was finally home! My surgery healing was underway, and my infection was under control. I had to keep taking medication, and all kinds of doctors' appointments were scheduled in for me. After all, I had to start chemo soon. Being at home was awesome even though I was still in pain. The home nurse visited me and put me on a course of antibiotics for another 10 days. It was about a week after my second unplanned surgery when I learned to take it easy. The removal of the Staph infection and the replacement of the expanders in the left breast taught me that my only schedule now should be to rest, sleep, eat, and drink fluids. I had never felt so weak, not even after the double mastectomy. I needed to fully recover from this surgery now, which had set my treatment back. A home care nurse would treat me until I was recovered. Dr. Bajnrauh would see me again the next week, and I would see my chemo doctor, Dr. Kato. I had surrendered to help and was accepting it with a joyful heart. I attended a follow-up appointment with Dr. Schroeder, and she checked on my Staph infection. It took a while to heal from that, and my antibiotics were extended to the 18th.

On February 12 I had my weekly follow-up appointment with Dr. Bajnrauh. I was feeling much better and was now off the powerful pain medication they had me on. Now I only needed to take Ibuprofen as required. The doc gave me a pep talk, and we talked about the emotions that I was going through. It is common to move through phases of difficult emotions when you have cancer or a challenging condition. You have to release and let go of that worry.

Dr. Bajnrauh removed one of the two drains and was pleased with my healing progress. He slightly inflated my left expander as well. I was taking it one day at a time at this point and continued to feel amazed at the support I was getting from friends and family.

The following day, I had my appointment with my oncologist, Dr. Kato. We chatted about the post-surgery findings—my one tumor was 5½ cm. The other tumor going into my muscle wall was smaller, about 2½ cm. The chemotherapy treatment plan had four sessions, one every three weeks. Treatments would be done at Dr. Kato's center, and each time a follow-up Neulasta shot was needed to help with white blood cell count the next day.

Blood work would be done each week, and my training appointment was scheduled for the 17th. I was told to expect information on the medication I would be taking and the sessions I would be having. Side effects were discussed, and they were scary.

A week after my antibiotic was finished, I would start chemotherapy. The next day it all hit me like a freight train. The journey that stretched out before me made me numb. I had a full diagnosis and treatment plan, and I knew all of the side effects I was to expect. I would have to have a CT scan that morning, a one-hour chemo class on Monday, and four 3–4 hour chemotherapy sessions every three weeks. I had to expect total hair loss, nausea, intestinal problems, and finger tingling.

Dr. Kato suggested that I cut my hair short so that I would minimize alarming the boys when it all started to fall out. Once my hair started falling out, my hairdresser would come to my home and shave the rest off, surrounded by my close friends. It was a lot to take in.

It is true that these things happen suddenly and discreetly. You do not really have time to stop and think. On Valentine's Day, February 14, Kathleen took me for a CT scan ordered by Dr. Kato. By the time I got home, however, the chills and fever set back in. I immediately called Dr. Bajnrauh and the home nurse. The home nurse came over, and both he and Dr. Bajnrauh instructed me to report back to the emergency room.

Jim G. and his wife Cissy took me to the hospital. Judi stayed home with my boys. Once I was admitted and given medicine, the fever subsided. Later on that evening, however, the fever came back, and my body just crashed. Dr. Schroeder and Dr. Bajnrauh handled my case. The PICC line would be removed, and more lab work and x-rays were performed. The root cause of my infection will need to be found. After two days in hospital, I felt stronger so they let me go home. I had to reschedule my chemo training while I tried to sort out this cause of the recurring fever!

Being at home was great, and without the PICC line, it was even better. I could shower without pain or nausea, which was a gift. I spent most of my time in bed resting. I ate dry food, water, and PowerAde for breakfast and kept it down. Lab results of the blood cultures and PICC line takes 72 hours—the doctors still did not know the cause of my infection. The following day I met with Dr. Schroeder—all tests were negative, great! I had no infection in my bloodstream. Since the tests and x-rays were clear, she concluded that I may have had a bad reaction to the contrast inserted into my veins for the CT scan.

The news was great—no more antibiotics or lines needed. Chemo was pushed back another week to give me time to recover. Later, when I saw Dr. Bajnrauh, he was smiling broadly. I looked a lot better than I had in the hospital over the weekend. He removed my drain so I no longer had any foreign objects attached to me. Now I had to focus on regaining strength. The next morning I was going to get my hair cut. This would be one heck of a journey.

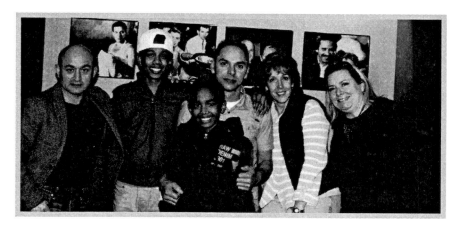

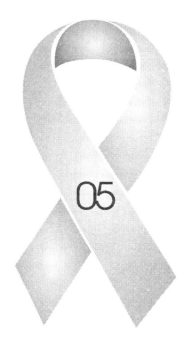

05

Taking
Chemo Classes

"As your faith is strengthened you will find that there is no longer the need to have a sense of control, that things will flow as they will, and that you will flow with them, to your great delight and benefit."

EMMANUEL

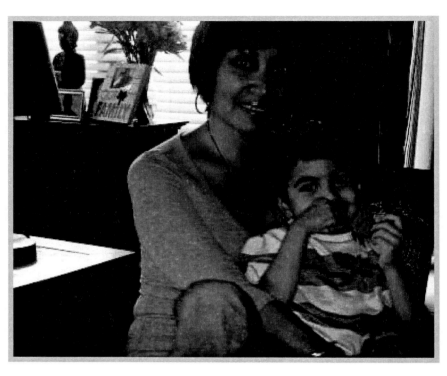

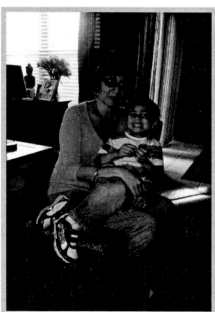

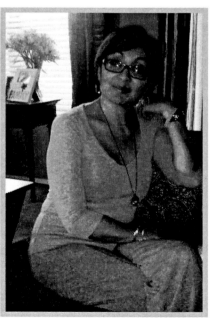

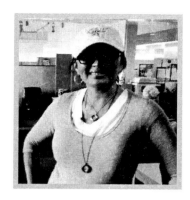

On February 20, 2014, I had my first haircut. My hair stylist, Heidi, was so gracious to come to my home. She cut it short. I had not had my hair that short since I was a teenager, and it would take some getting used to! Heidi did a great job, as usual! My hair would only get shorter and shorter from now on.

I had my first chemo class a few days later. Linda and Carla, my new Pink Sister, came along. Carla was diagnosed with the same condition some two years prior and had already undergone chemo and radiation therapy. We chatted and shared experiences, which was very uplifting. I did not feel scared or anxious like I thought I would, and there was a lot of information around to keep me reading. Instead, I chose to be optimistic.

The nurse outlined our care protocols during chemo and beyond. I recommend that you read through chemocare.com if you want a detailed rundown of what will happen to you. We got to see the room with recliners where the sessions were held. As long as I had a recliner facing the door, I would be fine. I hated having my back to a doorway. My first session was scheduled in, and I was told it would last four hours. I was eager to get started and to stop my cancer as soon as possible.

Waiting is always the worst part of going through something new, and I did not want to wait anymore. I saw Dr. Bajnrauh again; he is so kind, caring, and funny. They noticed my new haircut, which was great. The doctor was pleased to see my progress; I had recovered well from the previous week's events. He was finally able to perform expansions in both breasts during the visit. I discussed my chemo treatment plan with him, and we decided that he could only continue the expansion when my white blood cell count was high. The week before the next chemo appointment would be appropriate. I had been feeling really great for a few days, but I knew it would not last. I was taking it easy but enjoying the happier days.

On February 28, after feeling wonderful for a few days, I met with Dr. Schroeder for my final appointment. The blood tests that I had showed no evidence of infection! I got the all clear to begin my chemo. The bad news was that my liver was having problems. Before the Staph infection, I was okay, but the powerful medication I had been on had impacted my liver. Dr. Schroeder suggested that I drink a lot of fluids over the next few days to flush it out. Then on Monday I would have more blood tests. Dr. Kato would then need to review the results and decide whether I could begin chemotherapy. I decided to be optimistic and to embrace Dr. Schroeder's advice. So I went wig shopping! I had no idea what to expect, but I was excited to go.

Trying on wigs was a silly, wonderful experience. The store clerk was understanding and kind, and we all laughed together as we tried different styles on. It was a great moment, but wigs would take some getting used to.

By March 3 I was focused on being optimistic about my blood test results so that chemo could begin on Wednesday. I re-read all of the instructions, and the countdown to the big day began. Judi, Linda, and Jessica had arranged to ferry me to and from the treatment center, so that was sorted out. Gregory wanted to be with me the entire time—all four hours of it—so it would be a learning experience for us all. My mind and body were strong, and I was ready for the challenge.

By March 4 I was still waiting for the test results to check on my liver enzymes. Dr. Kato's office called me and asked me to come in for a retest, which I did. Monday's test showed extremely high enzymes, although the doctor suspected that might be an error. I reported to the lab and was in and out in 15 minutes. Hopefully, if the test was accurate, I could start my chemo—but if my liver enzymes were still too high, it would be a no-go. Chemotherapy can further damage your liver and lead to serious complications, so this was something we needed to check. I felt great, though, and was drinking aloe and coconut juice often. I even caught up with paper work!

The day came for my very first chemotherapy session. I got a call from Dr. Kato's office that my second test had shown my liver enzymes were far lower than the previous test had shown. Good news! I could begin chemotherapy. Finally, I moved into the next phase of my cancer treatment. I had taken the medication I was told to take the day before, and I reported for my first session. It was a piece of cake! I felt nothing at all out of the ordinary. I was started on Benadryl, which made me slightly drowsy. Gregory, Linda, and Judi were all with me.

Gregory listened to music and played video games throughout most of the time. I ate a giant foot-long sandwich and drank a bottle of coconut water. I even ate some of Gregory's chicken wings and fries. My appetite was great, and I felt nothing from that treatment. Jessica came and drove us home, and I modeled the wigs for her when we got inside. I started to feel quite tired and took my medication as instructed. I have to go back tomorrow to get a Neulasta shot to boost my white blood cell count.

I have to take a combo of Claritin and Aleve to prevent bone pain until my next treatment. There was also prescribed medication for nausea that I could take as needed. The next day was day 9 of feeling great! I continued to make the days count. I took a nap, ate dinner, and woke to another doctor's appointment with Dr. Kato. I had the Neulasta shot to boost my white blood cell count and left the offices feeling good. I kept my head up high and smiled with one chemotherapy session down. The boys were doing well in school, and I was having a particularly excellent day. Optimism can do a lot for your body I believe. The weekend was not as easy. Suddenly I experience extreme bone pain in my neck, back, and arms. The medication barely helped with the pain, but doctors told me the pain would not last. I struggled to sleep and move after that. The chemotherapy illness was upon me.

The bone pain was intrusive and kept me bedridden the entire weekend. The oncologist's office was not being shy about the pain; it was bad. I could barely move for a long time. On top of the bone pain, there was a headache, heartburn, and a deep feeling of frustration. When this happens, all you can do is wait for it to subside. Finally, I knew what to expect after my next chemotherapy session and white blood cell shot.

As you recover, you inch closer to your next appointment, which is why it gets tough. I had my follow-up appointment with Dr. Kato a week later. He went over the results from my CT scan from a month before that. There were minor issues with my liver, kidneys, and lungs but nothing too bad. We scheduled another CT scan for six months down the line. My liver enzymes were once again extremely high, but this is normal after a Neulasta shot. The pain eventually vanished, and I became upbeat and energetic again. I told Dr. Kato that the medication did not help, so he moved my chemotherapy session up a day so that I could have three shots (Neupogen, Neulasta, Neupogen)—one a day until Friday. This was set to reduce my pain.

A healthy diet and light exercise were recommended to keep me going, along with not gaining any weight, which can cause issues. The next few days were great; I felt no nausea, and my appetite was excellent. More than a week after my first chemotherapy appointment, I still had no side effects. I spent time walking, being productive, and running errands around the house. It had been Spring Break, so the boys were home with me, which was awesome. Gregory got his driver's permit, and I started teaching him how to drive. My next appointment was on Wednesday, so I made sure to treasure the time I had when I was not feeling terrible. I was ready for my next chemotherapy session.

At that point, I had been "home" for two and a half months. I felt well enough for a relaxing getaway from home, so we went to Bear Canyon in the Tucson Mountains. We walked a short trail, and I enjoyed the beautiful outdoors. I got some exercise and made sure that I kept getting stronger. I also stayed away from large crowds to prevent germ exposure. When it reached two weeks since my first chemotherapy appointment, I had still not experienced any side effects—no nausea, metallic food tastes, intestinal problems, hair loss, or tingling fingers.

My mind, body, and soul were doing extremely well. My appetite was ferocious, and I felt normal. I did, however, continue to take it easy. This is key to chemo because if you do not do it, you suffer.

The "new approach" to chemotherapy in session two would start the next week. I hoped that the new treatment prevented me from getting extreme bone pain again. Whatever happened I would keep my head held high.

The next morning I had spoken too soon. Each day my boys would joke and pull my hair, saying, "Nope, not yet!' but today was different. I had a strange sensation on my scalp, and there it was, a handful of hair. I did it again and again. Then I called the boys to show them—complete silence.

Reality hits you whether you are prepared for it or not. Losing my hair was disturbing, but I dealt with it. We all did. There is a sense of losing part of yourself, but you cannot let that weigh you down. It is, after all, just hair. It is not like your arms are dropping off. Take it in stride. During the process, I learned that sharing the experience makes it easier. Do not stand there and freak out alone. Grab a wig! My follow-up appointment with Dr. Bajnrauh went well, and he was pleased with my expanders and the stretched skin. He expanded them a little more and set the next appointment for three weeks from then. So, on the one hand, I lost all of my hair, but on the other, my expansions were going great.

Going bald is weird. I found myself in bed all morning pulling out my hair in clumps. I admit that I moped because of it. I always loved my hair; it was a huge part of my identity. I preoccupied myself with what I should do—shave it off or leave it? I called my Pink Sister, Carla, to ask. I wanted to shave it all off. I had already made up my mind, but I needed someone who had been through it before to validate it for me.

As soon as Carla's hair started falling out, she had her husband Nate shave it off. I made the bold decision to do it myself, and so I did. It was liberating in a lot of ways. It was a significant moment, like a spiritual ritual that needed to be performed. I did not cry or feel shock or sadness. By doing it in my own time, on my own terms, I made it a positive experience. Tye saw my new look when he got home from school first that day. His eyes and mouth were wide until he smiled. Gregory's response when he saw me was "Whoa!" I had not even thought about wearing one of my new wigs yet. My youngest son Liam yelled out to me, "Mom, you are bald! Now you can wear those girl wigs. Your hair will grow back. You are a winner!"

I am normally quite vain about the way that I look, but now I felt liberated and at peace. This liberation helped me take photos to show my family and friends and share on my website…but not right away. I had to adjust first. The day after shaving my head, I had to put together my new look. I started with the scarf, which gave me strength. My hair would grow back; I had nothing to worry about. Then, on March 23, I was hit with fatigue. I had to get out of the house to do some grocery shopping with Gregory. Because of that, I had to sleep all day the day before, all night, and most of that day.

Kathleen created an herb garden for me while many of my other friends worked in our back garden. The boys helped too. The whole experience humbled me, and I became extremely grateful for everything. I still cannot express what it meant to have that kind of support. So many people were looking out for me in a place where I had no extended family. I was full of thanks and glad to be healing!

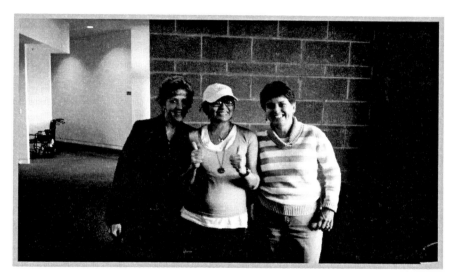

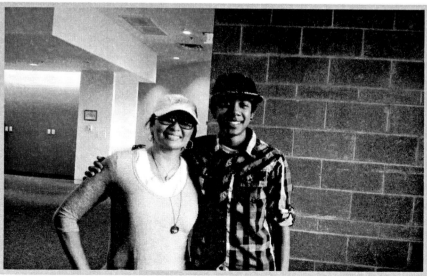

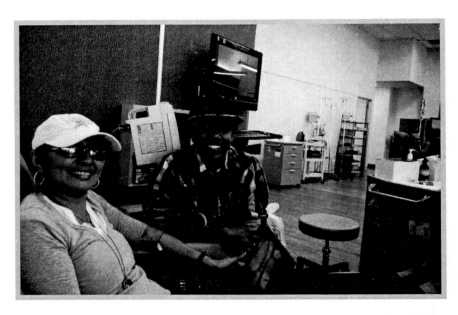

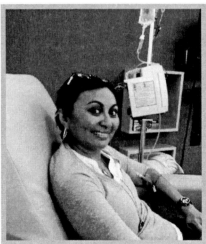

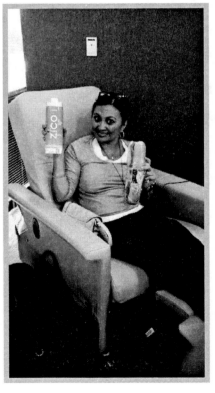

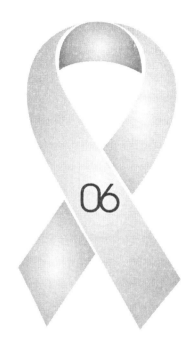

06

The Impact of Chemo

"When the Japanese mend broken objects, they aggrandize the damage by filling the cracks with gold. They believe that when something's suffered damage and has a history it becomes more beautiful."

BARBARA BLOOM

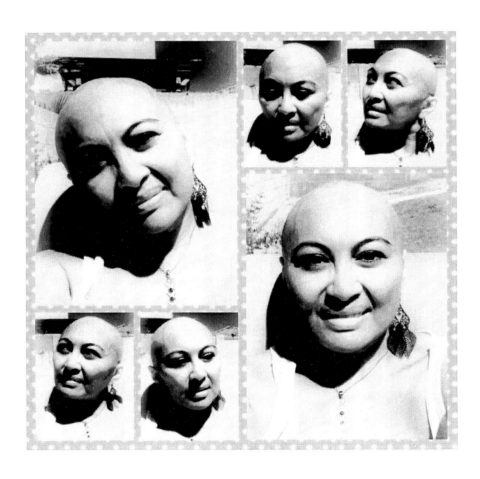

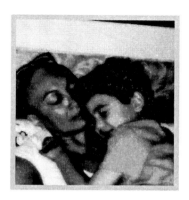

Being bald, I learned that my looks do not define me. I became adamant that I would continue to teach my boys courage, strength, patience, and endurance in the face of illness and challenges. That is what ultimately defines me! I wanted to get through this and live to see better, healthier days. It became my duty to do everything possible to survive this cancer.

Chemotherapy makes you feel like you need to overcompensate for the distress. My second chemotherapy session came, and Kathleen drove me there. She stayed with me until the fourth hour. Judi arrived during the final hour to take me home. Later that evening, I realized that the second session would not be like the first. I started to feel ill and expected another side effect like intestinal issues to crop up soon, which they did. I could not sleep until 2:00 a.m. that morning.

The next day the intestinal issues continued, although at a greatly reduced pace. I felt tired and unsettled, but I had to go in for my shots. A nap after my first Neupogen shot was not enough. I immediately went back to sleep. The next day, and again on Friday, I went for the other shots. Altogether I had three, along with the Claritin and Aleve to reduce the bone pain. I hoped that this change would result in less bone pain than the first chemotherapy treatment. The days had become harder, so I had resorted to taking each day as it came.

By March 28 I was very tired and worn from the shots and chemotherapy. I woke up one morning with stomach pain, and food started tasting off to me. Then I felt some pain in my lower back. I hoped against all hope that the pain would not return as furiously as it had after my first chemo session. Sleeping became difficult, and I realized that I was in the deep end. Despite my pain and struggle, I continued to look after myself and be positive.

When March 30 came around, I was feeling better. Dr. Kato's adjustment with the three shots made a world of difference. I was in a lot less bone pain than before, which gave me so much cause to smile! I did feel some pain in my lower back but nowhere as severe as it was before. I could get out of bed and move around—great! My stomach upset even went away. Though food tasted like bits of metal, I continued to eat and drink to maintain my strength. I sat outside that day in the shade, and it was lovely.

My one week follow-up appointment was scheduled in for Dr. Kato on April second. My vitals were all good, but my blood labs showed that my white blood cell count was very low. The doctor gave me another Neupogen shot to boost my numbers, and I had to go in again the next day for another shot. I also had to take a seven-day antibiotic in case I got sick. Dr. Kato told me to expect a fever, which I should then treat immediately with the antibiotics I had. I had felt energetic, pain free, and well, so I did not think about it much.

With only two chemotherapy sessions remaining, I could return to work after that. My last chemotherapy appointment would be Tuesday, May 6. After this final session, I would take a four- to six-week break before my reconstructive surgery. Then, after surgery, I would do radiation treatments. In comparison to chemotherapy, radiation would be a piece of cake. For five days a week, I would do 15 minutes a day for six weeks.

April 5 was a relaxing, quiet day at home. I played and cuddled with Liam, but I felt very tired. I took naps when I could, and Liam took naps with me! Tye watched TV while Gregory got ready to attend the Highland Jazz Festival to support the bands performing there. I started getting used to my bald look and even posted pictures of myself on my website for everyone to see. It took courage, let me tell you! I was happy that chemotherapy was half done and that my side effects had not been too bad.

When you receive treatment like chemotherapy, it weakens your entire system, so inevitably I got a cold and my chest was congested. I even developed a cough. So I called Dr. Kato to find out if I could take some over-the-counter medication. He told me there was no problem doing that at all. I bought some meds, and they made me feel extremely tired, so watch out for that if you develop a cold.

As I was feeling sluggish, I remembered that I had never taken the medication that my doctor had prescribed me for nausea. Not one day had I experienced any nausea, not one little bit. I did not want to jinx it when I told my family on my website, but I was thrilled that so far this side effect had not impacted me. I hoped that my third chemo session would render similar results to my first two with no nausea to speak of.

On April 9 I had my follow-up appointment with the awesome Dr. Bajnrauh. The expansion of the skin where my breasts should be looked great. The left breast did need to catch up to the right one, however, although they were looking more even. The expanders felt hard, like bricks. My final expanding session would be on April 23, then these expanders would be replaced with breast implants sometime in mid-June.

Later that day I had a hilarious experience with a security guard. While stepping through the security line, the officer hovered over my chest area with a handheld metal detector. It went nuts! BEEP, BEEP, BEEP! The expanders I had inside me each had a small magnet in them to indicate where the saline solution would need to be inserted so that they could be expanded. The security guard raised his eyebrows and looked at me with a questionable facial expression.

I leaned in close and whispered, "Oh, skin expanders…breast cancer patient." The security guard hurriedly responded, "Oh yes! Proceed, ma'am, and thank you!" It was such a funny experience that was handled really well by that guard. First he must have thought I was concealing a weapon somewhere unmentionable before realizing that a simpler explanation was warranted. Great fun!

By the time Saturday came around, my cold was much better. Gregory and Tye were tired from studying for their AIMS tests at school. I took them out to brunch, and then when we all got home, we collapsed from sleepiness. The boys watched TV and played video games, and so did I. Sunday was a better day for me as I felt upbeat and energetic now that my cold was fully healed. We went out for breakfast again and took a nice walk through the flea market. One of my favorite pastimes is treasure hunting, and what better place than the local flea market?

Gregory drove us there, which was great because it was needed. Then we went to the store and back home again. Later I felt fatigued, and when I woke the next day, I could not function well. I slept while the boys were at school, until I had to pick them up. My third chemotherapy session was coming soon, and I had to be prepared for it. The next day came quickly, and soon my third chemotherapy session was over. I was extremely happy that I was so close to the end that the session was super easy. I knew the routine, and I did not feel a thing. Jessica took me to the appointment, and Judi drove me home. Again, I ate lunch and drank a lot of aloe vera and coconut water. All in all, I felt excellent. Now all I had to do was get past the Neupogen shots—all three of them. My hope, once again, was that these shots kept that enormous bone pain away. Returning to work had been postponed to after my last chemotherapy session on May 6.

Some two days after my third chemotherapy session, I felt perfectly all right. Along with Claritin and Aleve, I would only need another shot the next day to ward off the pain. My appetite had remained good despite the persistent metallic taste. I ran short errands, did minor chores, and even met up with Linda and Teena during their lunch hour. More than anything, I believe it was my positive attitude that kept the side effects at bay.

That weekend was a storm of pain. Unfortunately, the Neupogen shots did not seem to work this time around. That is how it is sometimes with chemotherapy—you cannot predict the outcomes simply because you were fine the last time.

By Friday afternoon the bone pain started taking hold. It increased rapidly until I could not move. The severe pain emanated from my neck and shoulders down to my lower legs. At the very same time my intestinal distress struck once more. This made the pain especially challenging because I was visited by frequent hot flashes and stomach upsets. I had already been pre-menopausal the previous year with hot flashes, but I had been treated for it. I had to stop treatment for that when I was diagnosed with cancer. I spent most of my time in bed with limited movement and difficulty sleeping. The air conditioner was cranked up until my room was ice cold. I woke to night sweats and pain but had hope that it would subside soon.

The weekend was painful, and now everything was harder. I ate and drank as much as I could, though now I did it because I had to. All food tasted bad. I felt exhausted and perhaps the worst I had felt up until that point.

The next few days passed in a blaze of discomfort and survival. The bone pain and intestinal concerns were very real. They beat the pain I had after my first chemotherapy session back in March. The doctor prescribed me more pain medication, which helped. My white blood cell count was at an all-time low, and I rose wearily for my fifth Neupogen shot. After the shot at the treatment center, I got home and went straight to bed. No calls, no messages—I could not manage them. The following day was better, I had an appointment with Dr. Bajnrauh. He told me I was looking great, and we chatted about the exchange from expander to breast implants.

Dr. Shukla, the radiologist, would assist with the implant surgery before radiation treatment. She was also on the medical board that discussed my case. The stats are better with breast implants and radiation than extenders and radiation, so we planned around it. My implants would be done in the same hospital where I had my mastectomy. I had no more expansions because my immune system was so low, and the infection risk was too high. I left feeling cheerful about my new breasts.

Before I could settle into the idea that chemotherapy would have an end and I would get a new set of nice boobs, I had to go through another unexpected side effect. On Thursday afternoon hives began to pop up all over my body, from head to toe. I could not get any sleep with them. I took Benadryl, but it did not work. By Friday morning I had a fever of 101.6°F, so I called Dr. Kato and was told to head to the nearest ER immediately. I phoned Judi, and she blazed over and took me. They admitted me and ran tests and discovered that the pain medication I was prescribed was causing the reaction. I was treated with antibiotics once again—a different dose of Benadryl and Tylenol—and slowly the hives vanished. I felt better!

Late that morning I chatted to another doctor about my condition and mentioned the intestinal problems as a side effect of chemotherapy. He ordered my next stool to be tested and just as well because I had yet another infection. It was called C-diff and was highly contagious. (The average human digestive tracts is home to as many 1,000 special microorganisms. Most of them are harmless—or even helpful—under normal circumstances. But when something upsets the balance of the organisms in your gut, otherwise harmless bacteria can grow out of control and make you sick. One of the worst offenders is a bacterium called Clostridium difficile, a.k.a. C-difficile or C-diff.) I was placed in isolation, and everyone around me had to wear special robes, masks, and gloves.

My boys were not allowed to visit me, which was not ideal. I was taken off antibiotics as they can cause infections. Without an immune system, I had to eat and drink a lot—but this had risks too. I could not defend from food-based bacteria. I had to meet with another doctor to discuss an extended stay in the hospital for my own safety. I was fighting and staying positive. I hoped it would be resolved before my next chemo session.

The medical team treated me the next day, and I healed quickly. I was taken off the contagious list! A CT scan showed that I had kidney stones, but I was not in pain from them. I slept and waited on my blood results. Throughout the experience, I just wanted to recover and see my boys. To do that, I had to stay strong and fight through the infection. I did.

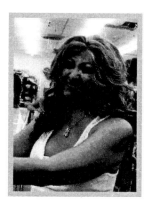
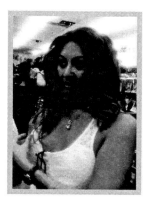
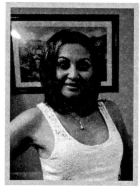

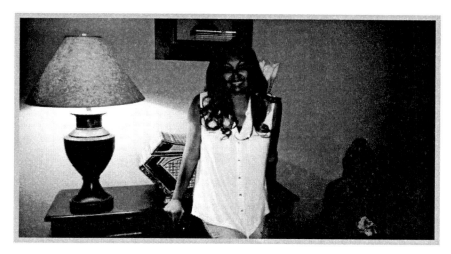

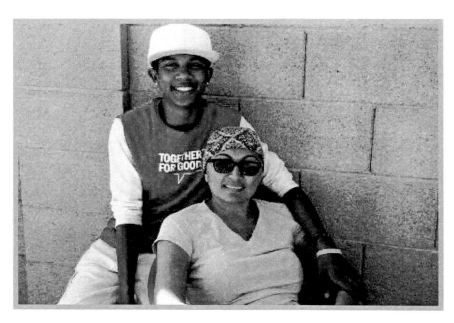

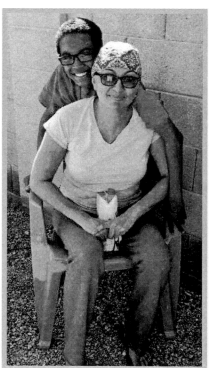

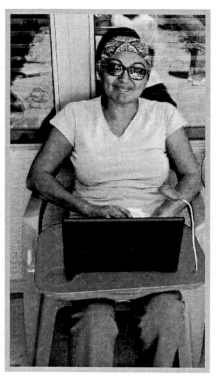

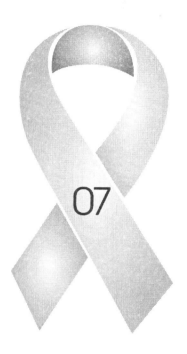

07

The Final Count Down

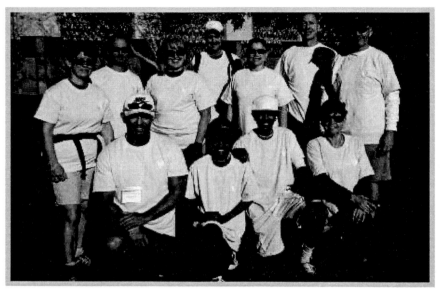

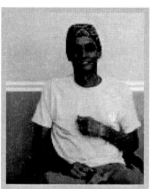

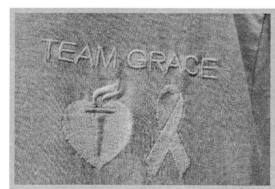

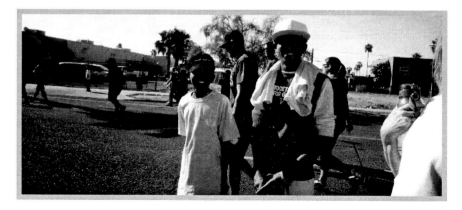

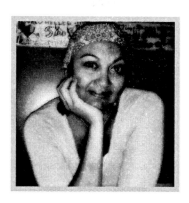

April 29 spun around, and I was brimming with emotions—with prominent moments of ups, downs, and tears. I was happy to be back at home, but the emotions of what was happening to me were taking their toll. Cancer is such a monster and one that you would not wish on your worst enemy—yet I was living through it. It changes your life to such a degree even though it is only temporary. Things that were so important before do get put on hold. I used to be so active with my boys, and we would come and go spontaneously from the house. While this year I was unable to participate in the annual 5K Heart & Stroke Walk, some of my fellow co-workers/family-friends participated in this walk and still included me by having formed separate team, even had pink t-shirts custom made with "Team Grace" on it as their way of support and brought Gregory and Tye along. I was incredibly touched, felt loved and honored!

I spent a lot of time reflecting on my life, my family, and my childhood that day. I had so many reasons to keep fighting this battle, and I would never give up. I had no pain but also no energy. My final chemotherapy appointment was in a week. The day after that was rougher than usual. I just did not feel right—I woke to chills but no fever. My eyes were itchy and puffy, and I was anxious about my future.

Dr. Kato called me in to check me out. He went through what happened in the hospital with me again and told me to stop taking my hospital prescribed medication. My blood counts were checked, and my blood pressure was normal. When the results came back, my counts were normal too. I was given additional medication to help with the overwhelming anxiety, which worked immediately. I was also put on an IV of fluids and slept for an hour—I felt much better after that.

The doctor told me I was still showing signs of the C-diff infection but that it was not contagious for my friends or family. Because of these rough days, Dr. Kato said that I may have to reschedule my final chemotherapy appointment. I was not happy about that, but in survival mode, I accepted it. I planned to spend the rest of the day resting, but not having someone at home to talk to was taking its toll. Cancer is ultimately a lonely disease, and without support, your days tend to grow darker.

On the second of May it was officially a week since I had been admitted to the hospital. Aside from the week I had that awful Staph infection, the past week was by far the worst I had suffered since being diagnosed. After another visit with Dr. Kato, I was living moment to moment, caught in the struggle. I could not keep any foods, fluids, or antibiotics down, which made treating the C Difficile infection really hard.

I had also developed a constant headache and occasional hot flashes. It was a sickening emotional roller coaster that I could not get off of. I ended up forcing myself to sleep with medication and woke at 4:30 a.m. Finally, I was starting to feel better! It began with my ability to keep crackers and water down, then an apple, and eventually the much needed antibiotics. I met with Dr. Kato, and he told me that I was doing better—and I felt it. He told me proceeding with chemotherapy that week would be a bad idea, so we moved the date. I spent another two hours hooked up to an IV, rehydrating. One of my nurses suggested Greek yogurt to help fight the infection. It had been a ferocious week, and I was very weak—changing, taking a shower, and eating were like scaling a 500-foot rock face.

The worst was over though, and the antibiotics took away the anxiety and headaches. By March 5 I was on the up and up and took the boys to school. Summer break was in three weeks, and I was feeling well rested. It had been extremely hot, with brutal summer heat meeting you wherever you turned. I needed to gain strength, and my infection was finally clearing up. I waited with bated breath on Dr. Kato's say-so as only he could decide when my next and final chemotherapy appointment would be. Hope was creeping back in, and my spirits were high.

The following day, I walked more to regain my leg strength, although I felt like an old lady hobbling around! I could not stand for too long, so sitting became an art form. I ate and drank and fought for quality sleep—my last day of chemo would come soon.

On May 9 my follow-up visit with Dr. Kato came around, and all of my vitals were perfect. It was a short appointment, and I looked and felt good enough for him to give me the go ahead for my final chemotherapy session.

Despite the weakness in my legs, we booked me in for Tuesday the following week. Dr. Kato reminded me that we would have to carefully monitor my progress after the treatment and three Neupogen shots. Each time the reaction had been different, but I was thrilled this was my last appointment. My final appointment would be the end of this segment of treatment and would usher in my reconstructive surgery—which I was very happy about getting. It was Mother's Day weekend, and things were looking up!

The day before chemotherapy, Gregory decided to join me again—he was there at my first and would be there at my last. I was so proud of him! Unfortunately, we found out that he had an important school test, which I insisted he study for. Instead, Justin would join me for the final four-hour long chemotherapy session. My leg strength was slowly returning, and I felt good. I was halfway through my cancer treatment and had renewed hope in my remission status, which I knew I could get.

Then, on May 13, the day arrived—my final chemotherapy extravaganza! The happiness I felt was close to indescribable. The session was quick, and that morning I felt strong enough to take it on. When it was over, my heart leapt for joy. I was two down (double mastectomy and chemotherapy) and two to go (reconstructive surgery and radiation). I was so happy with Justin's support on this significant day. After the three Neupogen shots the next day, on Thursday, and then on Friday again, I would be done. I chose to remain optimistic that they would help and not be as bad as last month.

Around 3:00 p.m. the exhaustion kicked in, and I went to bed. My mind that evening was filled with thoughts of my future and what life could be like again without cancer. To say my spirits were lifted would be a gross understatement. I even posted a video on my website journal.

The second day after chemotherapy, I was two Neupogen shots in and feeling good. I felt apprehensive about the next few days as I anticipated that debilitating bone pain that I had felt the month before. The thought that it was the last time I would feel that sustained me, and I continued to strengthen my legs. I walked short distances, but normally again.

My energy levels were all right, and I enjoyed a delicious dinner with Gregory while Tye came home from a football camp. Liam would be coming home the next day, and I had missed him terribly!

I paid Dr. Le, my primary care physician, a visit and dropped off some cookies. The entire staff had been so supportive all throughout my Journey that I wanted to give something back. I had not seen him since my official diagnosis.

We scheduled my radiologist appointment with Dr. Shukla for May 28, when we would discuss the treatments and whether it would be localized to the tumors or over the entire chest area. I also had another expansion with Dr. Bajnrauh coming up and a final oncology appointment with Dr. Kato too.

May 18 appeared, and fortunately my bone pain had not been as bad as before. It was bad enough to keep me from standing, walking, and doing basic things, but as long as I rested in bed, I was okay. The bulk of the pain was in my lower back, neck, arms, and legs. I took Aleve for the pain every six to eight hours and Claritin once every 24 hours. I was not complaining though; it was much better than last time! I ate and drank well, even with the intestinal issues that persisted. The hot flashes woke me at night, but I dealt with the frustration of it all.

Then something incredible happened—on the 19th I woke with no pain at all. I was a little sluggish, but it was an outstanding day. Not a single drop of bone pain! I only had some abdominal discomfort, and that was cake. So I stayed inside and caught up with some paper work. I was careful not to overdo it, but I did dance to some of my favorite tunes. The next phase was in full gear, and I was elated.

It was exactly a week after my last chemotherapy appointment, and I felt like Rocky Balboa at the top of the stairs. No pain for days! This was cause for a permanent smile on my face all day long. I celebrated in true Gracie style by splurging on a Cornish pasty, which is filo pastry filled with steak, potatoes, swede, and onions. It is an old English pastry dish out of the 13th century. My favorite! I felt compelled to celebrate this excellent day in a casual, student-like place similar to the pubs of my youth, when I studied back in Holland. The Cornish pasty near ASU was the closest thing I could find, and it had a decent European vibe with great music. I was the "Queen of Chemo," and I wanted to celebrate!

Schools were closed and grades in, and class parties were making their rounds with the boys. I was proud that no matter the circumstances, Tye and Gregory always achieved their goals. Tye graduated to freshman from junior high, and Gregory as a junior in high school. I was pleased as punch and proud as a mom could be.

My follow-up appointment with Dr. Bajnrauh happened the next day, which was lovely. We caught up, and I expressed my delight at being pain free. We discussed my surgery plans and did the final expansion in both breasts. The surgery was scheduled, and I would be able to go home the same day.

After surgery I planned to start working again. I could not wait to hug my coworkers and get back into the work vibe. May 22 was my follow-up appointment with Dr. Kato. I would not need any more chemotherapy or Neupogen shots, and my vitals and blood test results were perfect.

Now I only had the final two parts of my treatment left—reconstructive surgery and radiation treatments. I would not have to see Dr. Kato again until a week after my last radiation appointment. Pre-op and surgery were prepped with Dr. Bajnrauh for Friday, June 13, and Tuesday, June 17. I exercised every day and continued to strengthen my legs. I wanted to be nice and strong for surgery. The blessings from friends and family filled my heart. By May 23 I was able to go to work again and even attended my boss's team lunch that afternoon. It was an amazing start to a three-day Memorial Day weekend.

On Memorial Day, along with honoring those who fell to protect our country, I also focused more on leg training, which Dr. Kato thought would be a good idea. I had pushed myself to walk more and had gradually felt more and more upbeat. Once again I could do things like I could before—that feeling is incomparable. I spent time with my boys, chatting, singing, and laughing. I even tackled some staircases, though they took my breath away.

But I had pushed myself too far, and that evening my feet and legs were swollen. They looked like elephant feet. Carla, my Pink Sister, told me that my body was much more fragile than I realized and that I would bruise easily too. I had to elevate my feet and rest to make up for my eager attitude. The swelling went down, so I felt okay to go into the office the next day. When you have cancer, everything is different—and you cannot push yourself too hard.

Then the big day came—and I was back at work in the office. It was surreal sitting at my desk again, surrounded by my work family. I took the elevator and remained at my desk, but that did not stop my feet from swelling again. I elevated them and had a few visitors, so it was a very emotionally exciting day. I hugged, I laughed, and I cried—but the best kind of tears.

On doctor's orders, I took it easy, but it was tough to do that. On May 28 I had my initial consultation with Dr. Shukla, my radiologist. She was very friendly and took the time to listen and explain her treatment plan to me. Radiology would begin four weeks after my surgery with Dr. Bajnrauh.

My treatment would last six and a half weeks, not five, and each session would be 10 minutes long. We would have to see how my body would respond as the treatment progressed. It was my third day of work, and working from home was definitely the right move —I kept it remote and easy. My feet and legs were swollen again, so I kept them elevated. It did not matter though; I felt great. I was high from working again and had to prevent myself from catching up like a maniac, which was my first impulse. But I could not overdo it. Every hour or so I forced myself away from the computer and had my one-hour lunch break every day. I was productive and felt like a superstar once again.

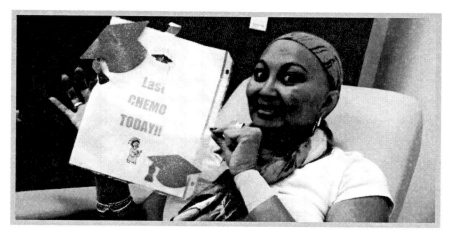

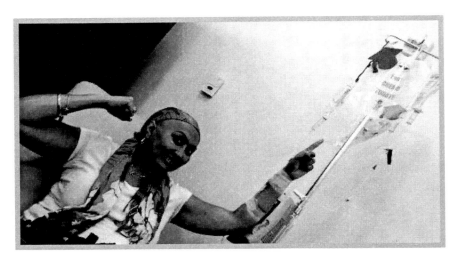

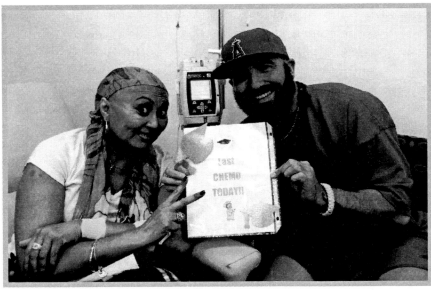

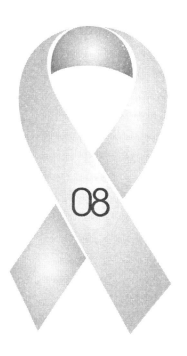

08

A New Pair
After Surgery

*"I can't change the direction of the wind, but I can
adjust my sails to always reach my destination."*
JIMMY DEAN

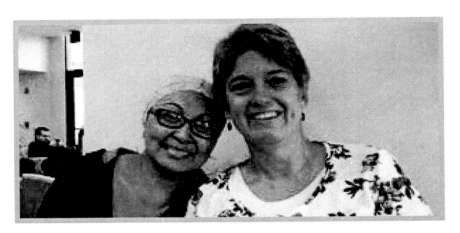

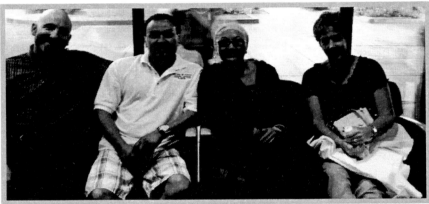

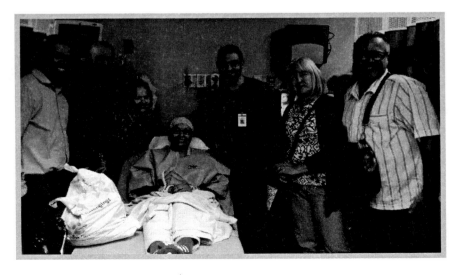

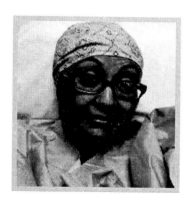

I was not sad to see chemotherapy behind me. That kind of experience is taxing beyond what you can read or what you are told about. With four whole days of work under my belt, I was getting work done and accomplishing goals. I felt well and barely experienced the effort. I focused on taking regular breaks and resting during my lunch hour—but the exhaustion would sneak up on me.

My body had been retaining a lot of water, and I felt bloated. I started taking natural diuretics, which helped. I had to gain some weight during chemotherapy to get myself through it, so I was heavier than usual. At the beginning of my Journey, I only weighed 105 pounds after dropping a load of weight—my normal size is 118 to 120 pounds. I now weighed 150 pounds, and I did not like it.

Once the bloating was gone and the surgery was complete, I expected my weight to come down. *Relax! It is only temporary*, I told myself. I needed the strength to get through surgery and radiation treatment. Food tasted normal again—no more metallic taste! That was a nice change. My plans for the weekend were to keep my feet up and cuddle, chat, and play with Tye and Liam while Gregory was on a much-needed break. He had gone to a friend's house for a sleepover dinner, and I hoped that he enjoyed it. Unfortunately, I did not have energy to take the boys out in public, and I wanted to avoid exposure to germs (or risk getting yet another infection). That was good thinking as it was 105°F anyway, which was scorching.

By June second the diuretics had worked, and I did not have any more swelling, especially in my poor legs and feet. I was very happy about that! The weekend was relaxing and restful, and I was feeling more and more like my bubbly self. Eating and drinking was still important to flush the chemicals out of my body. I entered my second week back at work with gusto while still taking it easy. It felt so good to get things done again and to focus on something other than my cancer! A productive and warm week was behind me.

By June 4 I had waded through all of my outstanding emails and could begin work with a clean slate. I discovered some changes that I had to adapt to and learn to figure out, but this kind of thing happens in business. I still took it easy and was extra cautious. My legs and ankles began to swell again, so I gave Dr. Kato a call. He told me that swelling often happened after chemotherapy and that I needed to continue with the diuretics and drink lots of water. I elevated my feet, took breaks to stand, and focused on eating healthily. I also went to bed early to make sure that I got enough sleep, which can be a killer if you neglect it. I met on June 13 with Dr. Bajnrauh for pre-op and was cleared for reconstructive surgery that Tuesday. His amazing assistant outlined the process for me—surgery, recovery, and medication.

I fully trusted Dr. Bajnrauh; surgery would last about three hours followed by two hours in the recovery room. The expanders would be replaced with implants, and there would be no drains. The skin was already stretched, so pain, recovery, and discomfort would be minimal. If we had not done the expanders, it would have been hell, with the recovery lasting a very long time. This surgery brought me another step closer to the finish line. It also landed on my three-week "return to work" anniversary. I did not feel as tired as I had been that first week, and I was ready for any new challenge.

June 6 brought about work satisfaction, which greatly pleased me. Margaret Thatcher once said, "Look at a day when you are supremely satisfied at the end. It's not a day when you lounge around doing nothing; it's when you've had everything to do, and have done it." I felt that way after each working day, but I was glad for the weekend rest. I took the boys to Main Event, where we could bowl and play billiards or laser tag. It was a reward for helping around the house. While they played, I enjoyed a two-hour long manicure and pedicure—it was heaven! When I got back home, I did some basic chores and rested; my legs and feet were a little swollen too. I was productive at work and got a lot done—plus surgery would be soon, and that would be life changing once again. I was happier every day.

June 17 arrived and with it my surgery. I was met at Virginia G. Piper Cancer Surgery Center again by an entourage, with Judi, Linda, and Justin by my side during surgery and for the recovery period. Kathleen, Julie, Llew, Dean, and Randy also stopped by before I went in, and we spent the time cracking jokes and laughing together. I was pleased that my day had finally arrived and that I would get my boobs back! Everyone met Dr. Bajnrauh, and the surgery went extremely well, lasting three hours in total.

I was in the recovery room for about an hour before being sent home. That day I learned a lot about gracious acceptance, which is an art. Most people never bother to cultivate the art of learning how to accept things from others. It can be much harder than giving, but it allows the other person to express their feelings for you. I was grateful beyond words for my friends and the gifts they gave me. I spent several days recovering, and by June 22 summer had arrived. I was uncomfortable and tired but completely all right. Doctor's orders were to rest, and I followed them to the letter.

My boys did not expect much, and they were tremendously understanding and deserving of so much more than what I could give them. I was not in any pain, so I stopped taking the pain medication. My chest did swell, but the doctor said it would be like that for a few weeks. At the end I would have some nice looking torpedoes. And yes, I mean boobs! When I had a one-on-one conversation with Gregory, he revealed to me that he remembered the exact day and location when he suspected something was wrong with me. Cancer even crossed his mind. I kept the diagnosis from the boys until it was official. While grocery shopping, he noticed me touching my right breast, where the lump had been. When two people are as close as we are, one always knows when the other needs help.

My recovery could not have gone any better, and I felt hardly any pain. I continued my antibiotics and completed them as instructed. Sleeping was still a challenge because I had to sleep upright, which makes comfort nearly impossible. I felt tired, so I would snag sleep on and off during the day when I could. I rested as well as I could. I had a follow-up appointment with Dr. Bajnrauh on Wednesday, and I felt great happiness and relief after that. My surgery was done, and I only had one more step to go to beat this darn cancer. Radiation was set to begin in four weeks, and I was hurtling towards the finish line with a smile on my face. I had a day where my air conditioner died, so sleepless days followed.

The pain medication and antibiotics did help me cope with the high heat though. I began to examine myself in the mirror, and I still had very few eyebrows and a bald head. But then, a few days later, my hair began to grow back! The peach fuzz that covered my head was the best thing I had ever seen. It grew black at the back and white on top—a unique look but not one I wanted to keep. I could not believe that my surgery had been over for a week already, but I was glad it was behind me. June 30 was a power day of productive work. I felt no pain, but I did have some soreness in obvious places.

Otherwise I felt energetic and enjoyed a relaxing stroll through the flea market, which was still one of my favorite things to do. I had to stop once again because my belligerent feet were swollen. So I took the boys to the pool and lounged around on a wet towel instead, keeping my feet elevated. That night it was hotter than the sun, but my swelling went down. On Sunday morning I saw a riveting game from the soccer World Cup, the Holland versus Mexico match. Holland won 2–1, which was incredible! I am sure my friends in

Mexico Mauricio and Ricardo, will never forget that loss! That week I was pain free with a relaxing weekend—what more could I ask for?

I attended my follow-up visit with Dr. Bajnrauh, and both Linda and Gregory came along for good measure. It was the first time that Gregory got to meet him. The hilarious thing was that Dr. Bajnrauh introduced himself to Gregory as "Robert" while all the while Linda and I had been calling him "Doctor B"!

Dr. Bajnrauh was very happy with the shape and size of my breasts, and the scars had healed well since surgery. The stitches were still in, so before I used anything to further heal the scarring, I had to wait a few more weeks until they disappeared. Dr. Bajnrauh was impressed that I had stopped taking the pain meds and that I was making good progress. I did not need to wear the wrap around my chest area, which is just as well as it was very uncomfortable. The good doctor suggested a sports bra instead, so I bought two on the way home.

When I arrived home that day, I still worked for another four hours. I have always enjoyed work as it gives me a great sense of value and purpose. Going back to work was a real reward for me because I missed my work family and getting things done. When you are an active person like me, cancer slows you down a lot. Sometimes I thought that the frustration of inactivity and not feeling well was the worst thing in the world. During those times, you have to remind yourself that "this too shall pass." None of those feelings last forever, and when you purposefully focus on the more positive things in your life, you make room for active healing. I worked hard on my legs and diet, and I believe it paid off. Many cancer patients that work through chemo and surgeries struggle to snap back to good health. Even with my weight gain, I managed to stay positive and enforce the doctor's laws. I ate, I drank, and I never gave up on looking after myself. That is critical. You can have other people looking after you—but never forget to take care of yourself too. That is what counts with cancer treatment.

On July 10 I finally went with Judi to see my radiologist, Dr. Shukla. She told me that she believed we should radiate the super clav area, where there are lymph nodes above the clavicle bone. She also said that we should radiate the rest of my right chest area to be safe. It was quite a controversial decision because I did not have any evidence of cancer there.

She believed that it might be an area where the cancer potentially could return, so it was done as a precaution. We took the fact that I had been in for a double mastectomy into account, so the precautionary measure made sense to us. Dr. Shukla also said that she would limit the amount of radiation that would go to my heart and other organs by focusing on potential problem areas. She was concerned about the fluid that kept building up in my ankles when I walked too much or stood too long. So I was booked to see a cardiologist who would make sure that my circulation was all right. While at Dr. Shukla's practice, I did a CT scan without contrast. I was glad not to have contrast near me as it caused the Emergency Room visit the last time I had a CT scan. I was sore from reconstructive surgery, and having to keep my arms over my head for 45 minutes was exhausting, painful, and endless.

I also received three little tattoos made by radiation needles to make the locations for the treatment. The skin on my chest area was no longer numb, so I felt those needles, and they hurt! After that appointment, I went to see Dr. Bajnrauh again, and he removed my last two stitches. Only two creases remained that were uncommon, but he was confident that over time they would vanish too. Then, good news!

My taste buds returned to normal, and I tested them on the best "liquid gold" jalapeno cheese sauce that I had ever had on a burger. It was so good that I nearly cried! My favorite cheese tasted metallic while on chemo, which was horrible—but no more! My hair began to grow back at a rapid pace now too. It seemed to grow back at double the pace of normal hair growth. I have always had early grey hair, so coloring is something I have done since my mid-twenties. I was excited to begin radiation and close the book on this cancer treatment.

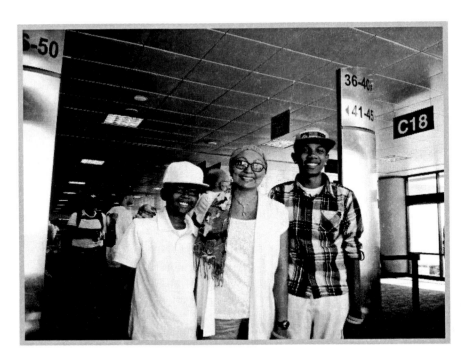

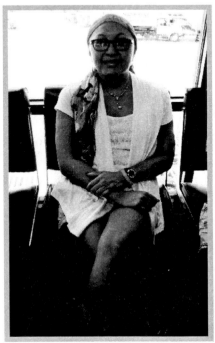

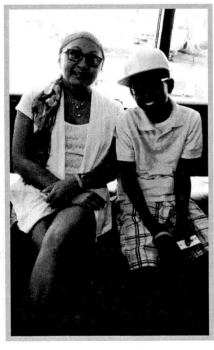

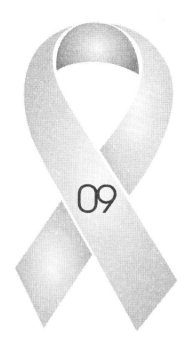

09

The Radiation Rodeo

"When you have come to the edge of all light that you know and are about to drop off into the darkness of the unknown, Faith is knowing one of two things will happen: There will be something solid to stand on or you will be taught to fly."
PATRICK OVERTON

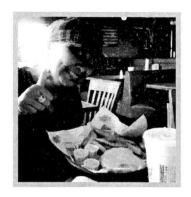

By the evening of July 10 my taste buds were almost 100% normal, and my hair was growing back again. I enjoyed indulging in my favorite food, jalapeno cheese on a burger and fries. Before, everything tasted like biting into iron! My hair was coming back with a vengeance at 1.25 centimeters a month, although it was mostly grey now. Soon I would pick out my new hair color—black, brown, or auburn—and it would be a brand new me.

The following day, on July 11, I had my appointment with the cardiologist. The swelling in my feet and ankles, I was told, was being caused by poor vein circulation or heart disease. To make sure that it was poor circulation, I was scheduled in for an Echocardiogram to rule out heart disease—scary! To keep the swelling down, I was prescribed Lasix, or Furosemide, and potassium, which would help.

The cardiologist booked me in for the Echo on July 23 with a follow-up visit on July 31 to discuss the findings. It had been a particularly tough week with my young son, so I decided to take it easy for the rest of the day. By the weekend of July 14, I was feeling more energized. I was lucky to be able to spend all of Saturday with my youngest son, Liam, at AZ Sea Life. It is an indoor complex and alternative to the more outdoor Sea World. The best news ever was that I was on my feet all day and did not have any swelling at all. I was a bit shaky up and down stairs, but the pain I had been feeling in my chest had all but subsided. On the whole, I had a great time! Now all I had to deal with was the pain on the right side of my shoulder and under my arm. I was very upbeat and energetic on Saturday and Sunday, closer to my old self than ever. With no doctor's appointments in the coming week, all I had to do was wait for my first radiation appointment. As for the swelling, I did not even feel like I needed the Echo anymore.

With a great weekend behind me, I called Dr. Shukla's office on July 16 to hear about the CT results and when I could finally begin radiation treatments. Imagine my surprise when she told me that the CT scan was normal and I could start radiation the next day! I was thrilled but nervous, as you would expect. Better to get it done right away so this experience could be behind me soon. I was told that I would have to undergo 33 radiation sessions. It takes as long as it sounds! My treatment would end on the first of September, or the second if the center closed for Labor Day.

I would be receiving treatment in three areas: my right breast where the tumors were found, under my right arm where lymph nodes were removed, and above my clavicle bone where more lymph nodes were situated. The little dot tattoos formed a kind of triangle, and we planned the treatments for midday to avoid traffic. I would have them done during my lunch hour and hoped that fatigue would not be too overwhelming. Each session was only 10–15 minutes long, so I would have time to eat, relax, and then get back to work. That was the plan anyway!

When I chatted to different people about it, I heard many conflicting stories. One person worked through the treatment without any trouble; another was hit with debilitating fatigue. So being an optimistic person, I planned for the best. Radiation is a preventative measure to extend your life span. The cancer was gone, but this would make sure that it did not return there. I was back in the office and happy to be there. Then the day of my first session came and went.

On July 18 I was hit with extreme fatigue. Dr. Shukla had to tape my left breast to keep it from being radiated as well, which took scan positioning and a lot of time to get right. The radiation room was pleasant enough, and they aligned the machine with lasers.

These lasers flash on the human body during treatment over the target areas. The top part of the machine moves from left to right over the chest area, and it does not hurt. In fifteen minutes, the actual session was over. Then the fatigue rolled in the next day, and I found myself unable to get out of bed. I dragged myself to my 11:45 a.m. radiation appointment and could only work until 3 p.m. The specialist said that symptoms only show up a week or two into the treatment, so I chalked it up to nerves and emotions running wild.

Having friends and family that supported me through this Journey ensured that I always got what I needed. Positive thoughts, prayers, and encouragement are like candy when you have had a bad day. I am still humbled by all the support that I have received. With the worst behind me, I finally realized that I was a survivor. That Saturday I slept all day and night while eating and hydrating in between—I needed it! I constantly had to remind myself not to overdo it, because my natural inclination was to do everything.

The Arizona summer was intense, and 30-minute drives to the radiologist's office were heavy. Each time I returned to the office for work. It was truly a day-by-day expedition. By July 24 it was tough to sleep and even worse to wake up. I usually wake at 5:30 a.m., but my days began slowly. I felt very tired even though the treatment itself was easy. I continually reminded myself that I was a cancer warrior and that this was the last stretch.

After each treatment, it was a step closer to freedom, an inch closer to health. I would not stop until I was done, no matter how tired I got. Nothing could slow down my progress! July 25 was a great day. I went to bed around 8:00 p.m. and slept all the way through to 5:00 a.m. A good night's rest totally renewed me! Another week's worth of treatments were behind me. I decided to change my treatments to be later in the day, at 3:00 p.m., so that I could beat rush-hour traffic and get home on time.

Honestly, the brutal midday heat was killing me, and I was not making it to 5:00 p.m. as I should have been. That weekend I planned to rest up, and that was it. My radiologist gave me a water bottle with the word "SURVIVOR" on it along with two rubber bracelets. One was grey, meaning "no one fights alone," and one was lilac, meaning "survivor." What a great keepsake for my radiation treatments on this incredible Journey. I was close to the end and desperate to get there! Only time was now on my side because I had already overcome the worst.

It is funny how time slows down when you near the end of a long, harrowing Journey. That is what it was like for me in those final days of radiation treatment—slow! I had done nine treatments and had 24 to go, and they could not come fast enough. I was very proud of how far I had come since my diagnosis and all the treatments I had endured and overcome.

The last six months were littered with setbacks, surgeries, unexpected fevers, infections, hospital admissions, and bouts of anxiety and depression, but as each hurdle came, somehow I managed to find my way back to myself—back to positive motivation and light. I began to feel like a true conqueror, something that living through serious trials can do to a person. I remembered my father's words at the beginning of this Journey—"Grace, no pity! Do all you have to do, and fight!" I had achieved this mission—I had won.

By July 31 this sentiment had sunk into my heart, and I was glowing! Then the exhaustion hit me like a truck. A UTI and kidney stone began to hurt me quite badly, and I realized the journey was not over yet. I took care of some work details then tended to my recurrent kidney stone issues. They always got pretty painful, but I saw my primary care doctor, and he prescribed an antibiotic to relieve the burning pain. Then I took some pain medication and drank a lot of water to flush out the stone. I napped for another two hours then headed off to another radiation session. Gregory drove me there and took me home again. It was great timing as he had just arrived back from a month's vacation in Florida.

When August 4 rolled around and the UTI and kidney stone issue was finally being sorted out, I was hit with a severe sinus infection. I woke to exhaustion and a sinus headache of note. I called my doctor again, and he put me on medication for that too. I had to call in sick and spend the day in bed; then I had another session. The long drive to the radiologists' office was tiring, but I had to be there, so I made the effort. I had no intention of delaying the treatments. The target areas began to look pink like I had sunburn, and the technician chalked that up to skin sensitivity.

The fifth of August arrived like a storm of fatigue, and I could only work for two hours or so before desperately needing to sleep. The afternoon arrived, and I was ferried off to my radiation appointment. The medication for my sinus infection cleared it up, and my treatment was quick and easy. The boys were back at school, so the daily routine has snapped into gear. I was 13 treatments in, with 20 more to go—nearly at the halfway mark.

By August 8 I was another week closer to the end of my treatments and the end of my cancer. With daily treatments, I had only been able to work for four hours a day, but I was making the most of them. It was my birthday in a week's time, and I initially wanted to host a big bash but then decided to wait until my final treatment phase was over. Then I could celebrate my birthday and my triumph over cancer all in one! My "family," as I call it (friends who are like family), would really enjoy a party like that. With all three boys in the house, it was the perfect time to do it.

The following day my right breast area was becoming tender and sensitive, and it looked like I had a bad sunburn. I used Aquaphor healing ointment, which is advanced therapy for dry, , and irritated skin; Dr. Shukla said that it works well, and I can confirm that it does. I visited Dr. Bajnrauh for a follow-up appointment, and he suggested I use more of the ointment than I had been. I spent a lot of time with my boys and took well needed naps in between the hustle and bustle of family life.

By August 13 I was pleased to find my hair was coming in thick and fast. I was halfway through the radiation treatments, yet my hair color still bothered me! Soon there would be enough to color. I joked with the radiation therapist that he must think he has a dream job being around boobs all day! We had a good laugh at that, which lifted my spirits. Skin "toastiness" is perfectly normal, according to Dr. Shukla, so I was on track. Tomorrow I would do a scar booster, which is extra radiation around the scars. Do not ever forget that a scar from cancer should be worn with pride.

I wanted to plan a big birthday party for Saturday but thought better of it—I just did not have the energy or strength yet. So I settled on the double celebration for after my treatment. I would feel much happier the next month when I was finally through this dark tunnel.

By August 14 I was suddenly struck with severe pain, and my friends Charlie and his wife Darlene rushed me to hospital. I was admitted, and the doctors ran tests on me all day long. Abdominal pain is the worst, and they could not tell me where the infection came from. I was given medicine and eventually diagnosed with acute colitis, or inflammation of the colon, the next day. The infection was chalked up again to C-diff, and I was given fluids, antibiotics, and pain medication through an IV. I slept and slept, all through my birthday. Just as well—I did not plan anything! The following day I was told to prepare for a colonoscopy and had to take Miralax all day without food. I never enjoyed days where I could not enjoy at least something to eat!

After my colonoscopy, I tested negative, so there were no issues there. I did test positive for a C-diff infection though, so I had to stay in the hospital until Monday. Because of my diagnosis, everyone that visited had to wear gloves and a gown—as before, I was highly contagious.

After the diagnosis, I rapidly improved and came off the IV. I ate real food and reverted to my old self! As the infection died, I felt stronger and stronger and even saw my friends as they stopped by. By August 18 I was only on oral morphine, and my appetite was back. Vancomycin put a stop to the C-Diff infection, and I used Saccharomyces B Florastor to restore good bacterial flora.

Once I was able to return home, my radiation treatments would continue—just another bump on the road to full health. The next day I was released, to my great relief. I arrived home a little before noon with an antibiotic and some pain medications. I was in a jovial mood, although I still tired very quickly. Now I had to call Dr. Shukla and Dr. Kato to reschedule my follow ups. Radiation treatments resumed on Monday! I was so happy to be home with the boys again, and as always, the thoughts and prayers made all the difference.

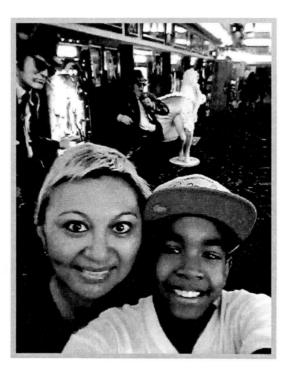

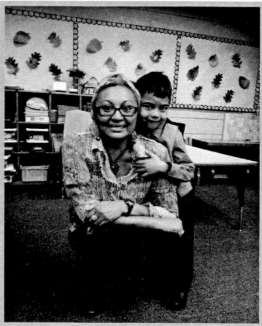

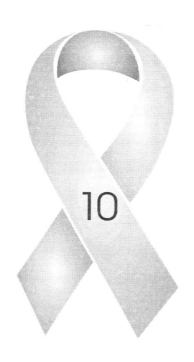

10

The Final
Countdown

"Remember, if you ever need a helping hand, you'll find one at the end of your arm ... As you grow older you will discover that you have two hands. One for helping yourself, the other for helping others."
AUDREY HEPBURN

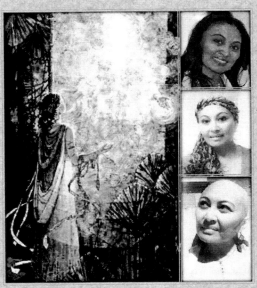

实力 "Strength"

There is no beginning or end
to your dreams and plans...
Life is a journey from moment to moment
The light within is not an illusion!
My determination, will and desire to
Live, Love and Laugh is real!
And nothing, you hear me?!
NOTHING will stop me from doing so!

~Gracie

勇气 "Courage"

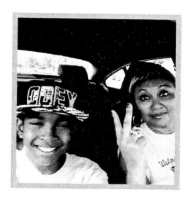

Being back home after another hospitalization was paradise. It was a very good morning for me waking up in my own house. For one, I had perfect, uninterrupted sleep, and I could see my kids whenever I wanted to. I did feel tired, though, so I took the rest of the week off. I would get back to working part time on Monday. With any luck, Dr. Shukla would approve the radiation treatments for then too. My birthday was lost to the hospital haze, but I had to let that go. Even though it is the most important day of a person's year, there was always next year! I have always embraced birthdays—growing older is a privilege. I received many birthday wishes from my friends and family, and they warmed my heart.

By August 22 I was back in the routine of sleeping, eating, and drinking—survival mode after the hospitalization. Nothing reminds you more about your mortality than a hospital stay. It was one day at a time all over again for me. The first time I actually left the house was on August 24 for some grocery shopping. It was wonderful to be out and about, even if it was only for an hour. I had to start all over again, with light chores.

I had become very forgetful, which was a challenge, and I had to keep my frustration in check. "It is just temporary," I kept reminding myself. The next day I would start work again for a maximum of four hours only. Then I would continue hurtling through the radiation rodeo. With optimistic thinking, I could get back on track and have no more setbacks. This was my final stretch. I only had 17 sessions left, and I was going to cruise through them like a hot knife through butter. I only needed to focus on my recovery and not overdo things. Plus, I had that wonderful double celebration to plan, which would mark the end of a very long journey. This was the final countdown, and I was so happy to be there. Nothing would chase me away this time!

I had a lot of catching up to do at work because I had missed the last week of it again! The good thing was that it helped pass the time, and I was happy to do it. Dean took me for a healthy and tasty lunch before heading off to radiation therapy. I felt an unusual muscle ache that stretched across my chest and shot up my upper right arm. This time it was painful putting my arms up when I was positioned for the session to begin. I made a mental note to mention this when I met with Dr. Shukla again later in the week.

On August 26 the muscle aches got worse, and my skin began to tighten uncomfortably. I chatted to Dr. Shukla about it, and she assured me that the pain was perfectly normal from the exposure to the radiation. It would hurt like that until the treatments ended. She suggested that I rotate and stretch my right arm as much as possible and use the Aquaphor cream more often.

My hospitalization caused the sessions to be pushed back by almost two weeks, so I was quite a bit behind. Now I had to figure out how many sessions I still needed with Dr. Shukla. She told that working half days was still a good idea through the entire month of September and maybe even longer—depending on how I eventually felt post treatment. I did not want any more setbacks, so I did not argue with her, no matter how much I wanted it to end and return to normal again. I was still due for my scar boost, which was interesting.

On August 28 the last stretch loomed ahead of me, but I felt like I had transformed into a sloth and was crawling as slow as humanly possible towards the finish line. Time was standing still! I did my work at the office and held short conversations with people, but I was still so forgetful. Then I went to treatment and off home, where I would sleep for the rest of the evening. All I wanted to do was sleep! I was determined to get through this very strange phase, though, so I kept at it. I was still excited about each step, and Labor Day was fast approaching. I looked forward to the last treatment of the week and the three-day break I would have in between sessions. I had no holiday plans, but the boys and I would watch a nice movie and have dinner out somewhere. Everything else was still rest and survival mode.

September 2 swept by, and the long weekend was flecked with bouts of minimal pain and that sagging, hovering tiredness I had been feeling. I needed to leave the house, so I went on a short road trip for the day to visit Joshua Tree National Park. Now that Gregory could drive, it was easy getting there, and the scenery was utterly breath-taking. The park itself was world famous, and I left the car a few times to drink in the surroundings and count my blessings. I strolled here and there, although hiking would have been fun. Sleep had become an issue as the pain, discomfort, and fatigue took their toll. Sometimes I had shooting pains in my breast area. So being out and about was much needed and a real healing tonic.

On September 4 I had that radiation scar boost I needed. This is when you are given a higher dose than routine radiation treatments, which target the tumor bed. The dose itself only covers a small area, where the cancer is most likely to return. These radiation boost sessions are usually given once routine treatments are done, but I would require five more boost sessions. These drastically lower the risk of recurrence in the same spot. I had experienced some intense pain on the left side of my breast, and when two of the technicians felt it, there was some kind of "knot" there. I tried to get an appointment with Dr. Bajnruah, but he would be in surgery all day. I did schedule an appointment with Dr. Shukla though, so that she could examine the area. I hoped that it was nothing serious and would be easy to resolve. When you go through this much for cancer, you just never know what lies around the corner.

Dr. Shukla was not in, so I saw another doctor. He believed that the pain was caused by nerves growing back in the areas that were cut during the operations I received. About two to three months later after major surgery, this tends to happen, so the time was right. I was not so sure about the diagnosis, so I decided to check with my other doctors anyway. In the meantime, I took ibuprofen and Tylenol for the pain.

At one of my radiation appointments, one of the technicians was kind enough to write down information about these booster treatments that I was getting. They are officially called "electron boosts." They only treat the area where the tumors were removed and the scar in that area. They were not for the scars after my reconstructive surgery. The rest of my breasts would start to heal, which I was happy about.

On the day of my first boost treatment, Dr. Shukla came in and showed me where they would direct the radiation. It is a complex process, but the doctors know what they are doing. By September 10 the pain on my left side had begun to subside. I told Dr. Bajnrauh anyway, and he confirmed that it was nerve pain—ouch! As the new nerves grow throughout the area of the surgery, the pain can be very specific to that location. After what I had been through, a little nerve pain was fine as long as it was normal. That was my final visit to Dr. Bajnrauh, who was leaving for LA. It was a sad last visit—on the one hand, he was happy with my healing and outcomes; on the other, I was sad to see him go. But LA was a great place for plastic surgery, so I knew he would be a rock star there.

Then Dr. Shukla decided to give me the best present ever—Friday would be my final day for these radiation treatments. Friday would be the day I could officially call myself a cancer survivor! Technically, you have to be cancer free for five years to claim that title, but according to Dr. Shukla, I could count September 12 as my official date of survival. After all of those trials, cuts, pain, bruises, and scars, I would finally be done. It may have tried to kill me, but in the end, I killed it first! Suddenly the day arrived, as suddenly as my diagnosis. I now love the number 12. Each year now I will celebrate the twelfth of September as the day I crawled over that finish line! It was my last radiation treatment, and I was in super high spirits.

Another bittersweet farewell, this time with the radiology staff, could not even get me down! Dr. Shukla, Darlene, Flore, Miranda, Amber, Ashley, and Rafael—I will never forget your attentive care and kindness.

My next appointment would be a follow up with Dr. Kato, my oncologist. I would have to take a pill, Arimidex (Anastrozole), an estrogen blocker, every day for the next five years, but I did not mind. My nightmare was over!

On September 16 I had a lot to do, and now that the treatments were behind me, I was quick to forge ahead—with my body suggesting otherwise. I had to remember that I could not do everything just yet, but it was so hard. I spent hours at the MVD, and Gregory passed his driver's test, now fully licensed! I had some car trouble and got it repaired. By mid-afternoon I had done too much, and I crashed. The rest of the day I was in bed, feeling regretful. The next day I could barely do four hours' worth of work, so I paid for it for two days afterwards.

By September 23 I saw Dr. Kato to discuss the new medication I would be on. He told me that I did not have to take the pills, but that research showed they did keep a lot of cancers away. Because of my double mastectomy, I would not get cancer there again, but it could come back in my lungs, liver, or bones. He strongly recommended it, so I agreed. The two types were pre-menopausal Tamoxifen and a post-menopausal kind too. Using a blood test, he would determine which type I was so that I could begin the treatment.

Tamoxifen is the one most commonly used, but it could cause hot flashes and blood clots in my legs. My family history suggested that blood clots would not be a problem however. If I was post-menopausal, I would be on one of three drugs. Then I would need to determine which side effects I could live with from the three. Hot flashes, bone pain, and a higher chance of getting Osteopenia or Osteoporosis would be in the cards. A bone density test would need to be done in this instance and one annually during a checkup.

Once we settles on a drug, I would need to see Dr. Kato in eight weeks' time, with my next appointment on December 19. Then it was just a simple matter of seeing him every three months for the first two years then every six months. If at any time I felt intense pain in my bones or struggled to breathe, I should see him immediately. I had also been placed on 1000mg of vitamin D and 1200mg of calcium.

Once the drug class was sorted out and my vitamin D and calcium levels checked, I was in very good spirits. I would see Dr. Kato again, so no sad goodbyes were necessary. My blood test results came through later that day when I received a call from Dr. Kato's offices.

It turned out I was post-menopausal, so I would be placed on a medication called Arimidex, which I would have to take every day for five years. My vitamin D readings were also very low, and that needed to be sorted out. A good reading is 30–100, and mine was 13! So I was prescribed 8000mg of vitamin D once a week for eight weeks at 2000mg a day. Other than that, my calcium stayed at 1200mg per day, and the rest looked great. I still needed to have that bone density scan before my December 19 appointment, which we scheduled in as I was in the post-menopausal group.

From September 28 onwards I was in full recovery mode. I had taken Arimidex for five days and was used to taking it first thing in the morning. I made an effort to walk more by not going straight home after working for four hours a day. Even though I was still tired, errands were good for exercise so that I could regain my strength. The next week would be my last of four-hour days, and then a full day would hit me again. I needed to be ready for that! It would be nine months since I last worked a full day, so I was excited and terrified at the same time. I did not want to overdo it and end up in the hospital again, but life does not wait for you forever.

Eventually you have to push yourself to re-join society after something like cancer. I hoped by that time my mind, body, and spirit would be ready. One day at a time was really the best that I could hope for. Every day still posed its challenges, but I was growing stronger and better with every passing week. Work is something I have always enjoyed, and reconnecting with my colleagues would really be something special. I had sorely missed many of them and the joy that they bring into my life.

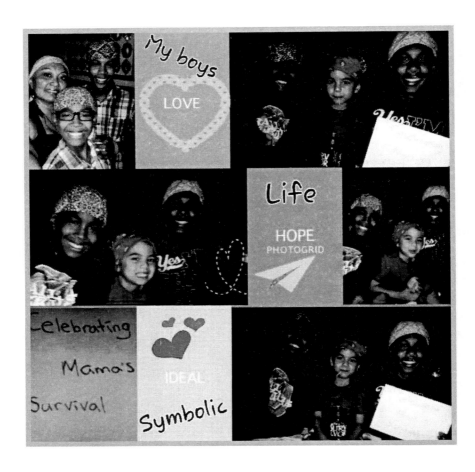

11

Recovery and Discovery

"Yesterday is but a dream, and tomorrow is only a vision, but today well lived makes every yesterday a dream of happiness and every tomorrow a vision of hope."
ANONYMOUS

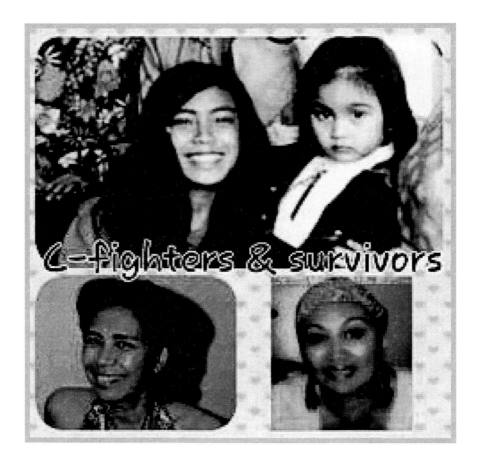

C-fighters & survivors

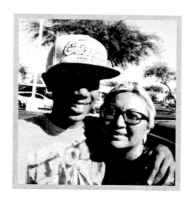

The worst was finally behind me! Then on October 1 I realized that the fatigue that had been plaguing me had gone away. Half the week had come and gone, and I was still full of energy. Honestly, I felt incredible!

Work was rolling forward like clockwork, and errands were becoming little things again. I had not taken a nap in three days, because I had not needed to. My appetite was excellent, and I got lots of exercise and hydration. For the first time in almost a year I was able to attend school concerts at my sons' schools, within a week of each other! It took a lot of energy, but what a life change! Seeing them there was the most wonderful feeling in the world. The boys were happy that I was back to see them experience life. It was Tye's first year in band, so it was a very special concert indeed.

I had been taking Arimidex for over a week with no side effects, although I had been told to expect bone pain eventually. Exercise would help minimize that, and as a result, I was walking as much as I could. This month was Breast Cancer Awareness Month and HIV/AIDS Awareness Month, so I was planning to walk in both events. From the next Wednesday, I would work full time again. I was easing my way back into the swing of things by working three full days the next week. If I started feeling too tired, I would have to stop and leave or risk health ramifications.

By October 9 I had experienced my first day back at work, and it felt brilliant! At the end of the day, I did not feel as tired as I thought I would. I even went to dinner with a nice group of friends. I took my hour lunch break and rested, and then powered through the rest of the day like a champion. I was glad that I was easing my way back in, so I managed to treat Gregory, Tye, and Liam to a short weekend road trip to Lake Havasu. They deserved it after the previous nine months of trials. Every day I gained energy and strength, so the trip was incredible for some R&R. Swimming was a challenge after the surgeries, but other than that, I coped well. The weekend came in a rush, and the feeling of accomplishment set in. The boys and I enjoyed a replica of London Bridge and an old authentic gold mine on Route 66 on our short trip away.

I was hit with another bout of painful kidney stones on October 16, which slowed me down a lot. I had a very important task at work and could not take the day off. So the day was a total challenge—but I rose to it! At the end, it was productive and successful, and all I needed was some pain medication to keep me going. At 4 p.m. I got home and napped immediately. The tiredness was caused by the pain, and I hoped the stones would pass soon. I have had these episodes many times before, and if the pain got any worse, I would be back in the hospital. There was no work the next day, but I was scheduled to volunteer at an LGBT luncheon.

October 20 arrived cheerfully with a week to go before a whole year had passed since I had first found the cancer lump. It was a relaxing evening after a full day's work when I rolled over in bed and suddenly felt a hard lump in my right breast. I was immediately alarmed as the lump was completely foreign and out of place. That lump kept me awake all night, and I was determined to be the first in line at my primary care doctor the next morning. From the age of 40 I had always been adamant about mammograms and had gone each year in April. The lump was not there then! It was six months later, and now I had a mystery lump. That is how fast it can happen.

I knew my body well and felt that something was extremely wrong.

On October 21 the bone pain I was promised finally arrived. It is the most common side effect of the generic drug I was taking. Exercise minimizes the pain but does not eliminate it. Some days were good, others were bad—but I was growing stronger. I would never give up on trying to attain full health.

I had been back at work for two weeks and was due to see Dr. Shukla again. I was feeling good, and the areas of radiation looked great; even the scars were healing well. My "big sister" Kathleen came along to listen in and take notes. I never really understood what the doctors told me; it was all so emotional and overwhelming. Writing recaps in my journal had been a constant challenge because of my memory problems too, so it helped to have someone else there.

The day came when I decided to tell everyone that I was turning my website into a book—something that can help other cancer patients orientate themselves in what might happen to them through my Journey and hopefully become inspired to fight back against cancer. I have learned so many lessons, and now I have this book to show for it. I cannot believe that I have reached the day when I decided to create a book, and now I have one!

By October 25 I was feeling on top of the world. Work started off well, but then—BAM—another reminder to take it easy—a panic attack! Apparently panic attacks are normal for breast cancer patients. I had a great lunch with friends and put it behind me then finished my work shift. When I got home, I was anxious again and could not eat. By the next morning I felt a lot better, and I had a great day with my middle son, Tye. We shopped together and found some good winter deals along the way. Then we saw a movie at a small local cinema, which was lovely.

Tomorrow I would take part in my first walk for AIDS in over a year! The 3.1 miles would be great to ease my bone pain. It would be my fourth consecutive walk. The next day came, and we set off for the 5k walk. I had strength and energy and did it with ease! What fun we had with nothing but big smiles and happiness.

To top it all off, October 27 arrived, the day I first discovered the lump. It had been exactly a year since the journey began, and I reflected on it. It was all behind me now. I had triumphed over it! I felt at peace for the first time in a long time. Most of all, I was grateful for the lessons I had learned along the way. Courage can get you through anything if only you are willing to find it inside yourself.

I greeted October 31 with love in my heart. I met the sun with love because it warmed my bones, and I met the rain with love because it cleansed my spirit. The third week of work was behind me, and it ended with accomplishment—I got a lot done. The last time I went on leave it was December 28 the previous year, and although it had been a large gap, the past week had felt like I had never taken time off. I felt overtired the previous afternoon and thought that I might not make it through the day. But I went to bed early the previous night and woke up feeling upbeat and completely energized.

Going to bed early makes all the difference. I am now hyper aware of limiting my stress levels by taking it easy and not taking on more than I can genuinely handle. I force myself to eat and drink well because those are the basic building blocks of life. It was a beautiful night, and the Arizona heat was dissolving into beautiful months of ideal weather.

November 2 was a very relaxing weekend. I needed the rest, so I kept activity to a minimum. I am glad to report that my bone pain was minimal too. On my bad days I take Aleve because it works better than Ibuprofen. Aside from that minor bump, I feel amazing. I am even considering joining a gym soon. I would love to focus on swimming, some light weight lifting, and perhaps even venture into the exciting world of Zumba.

November 7 marked the day I was officially diagnosed with breast cancer, so when it came, I had cause for celebration. Stage 3 breast cancer is no joke—what a Journey it has been! There have been so many tribulations, and now I do not even have bone pain. My medication is once again all right, and each day is better than the last. My health is rapidly returning, and I am well on my way to a full recovery. Life quickly returned to normal, although it can never be completely normal again. Working, kids, household, dogs, appointments peppered in between—I spend most of my time with my boys, who were giants through this experience.

It is funny how the most serious things in life force you to walk the hardest paths. And once they are walked, there is no turning back. Yet life goes on as it always will, and somehow you have to fit back in to a life you once had.

This book is my gift to the world and to other cancer sufferers—people going through what I went through. There is no describing the feelings that you feel when you are diagnosed. There is no "dealing" with cancer. There is only survival and fighting back, day by day. I am a Buddhist, and that means being self-righteous when doing things that make me feel good, doing and being good to others, and making others feel good about themselves. I have no judgment, only a powerful desire to teach, learn, inspire, and encourage those that face that dark tunnel ahead. At times it may seem too long to bear, too dark to find your way, but you must find a way. Respect for yourself becomes the most critical thing in life when you are diagnosed with cancer. Then, another challenge—a close family member was diagnosed with the big "C." How evil that foul plague can be! Now I must return the love, help, prayers, and support so that she can make it through the tunnel too.

On November 29 I could not rest from a challenging week. Work had become very busy, and I needed to prove myself all over again. I was being proactive and loyal and showing my work ethic wherever possible. My allergies were still causing me strife, and I had to report to urgent care for breathing treatment one evening. Again I had to take off work, but I would not let it get me down!

Thanksgiving had arrived, and I had a lot to be thankful for! This year we did a potluck, and it turned into the celebration that I wanted to have all along. Great food, great friends, and better laughs saw us through the evening, but these are really the things that see us through life, aren't they?

December arrived along with the usual festive cheer. I was back in full force at work, and the days were flying by. I have always loved my job, though I need to keep myself in check. It is easy to allow work to compromise my health, so breaks have become vitally important. I make a point of leaving the office at lunchtime to seek out life, which helps. Whether it is to run errands, to have lunch, or simply to take a walk, nothing is better. When I get home, my energy is low, so I eat quickly and spend time with my boys. Enough sleep is always a key priority. My bone pain is very little these days, just stiffness in the arm and knee joints if I sit still for too long.

Walking is still my main exercise, and it is all I can handle right now, but I am optimistic. I often wonder if I will ever get my full strength back, but I know it will take time. Everything takes time in the end, and cancer brings that into sharp focus. At my first quarterly visit with Dr. Kato, my oncologist, the bone density scan was normal—no signs of osteoporosis or osteopenia. This scan will be done again in two years. They did a blood screening, but I expect good news.

Doctors are now part of my health and my life, and I am better off for it. I wrote my final journal entry on December 28. I announced that my site would be taken down in January. Recovery is slow, but my spirits are the highest they have ever been. Cancer will impact everyone in this life, and I am convinced my story will do some good, even if it is just to let you know that you are not alone and to communicate the special lessons I have learned along the way. The next chapter is dedicated to those lessons, so do open your heart, your mind, and your spirit and consider what I say. The storm of life sweeps by quickly, and if you are not careful, you will be swept away too soon. I am eternally grateful to all of my supporters, friends, and family who helped me find a way out of the dark. I believe that you can find a way to free yourself of cancer too. Never stop fighting!

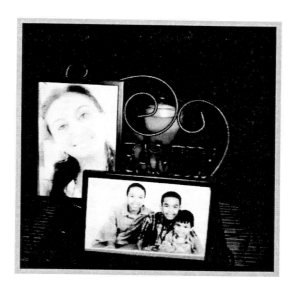

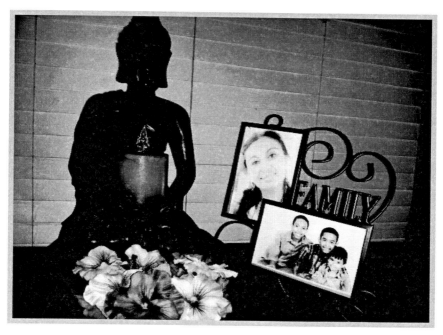

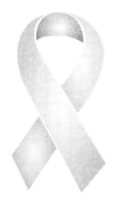

Closing Words:

A Note to Fellow Cancer Patients

I spent a year fighting cancer, and make no mistake, it is a fight; not the kind that happens on an obvious battle field but the kind that you cannot see. The only way to win this war that is raging inside your body is to make sure that you live for your health. That means taking precautions at every level to ensure your survival. It means— even if it is against your nature—to become selfish with your time and energy because there will be days when you will desperately need to care for yourself.

Cancer is unique in that it wants to kill you, so this is a life and death scenario. It is not good enough to just "do your best" and hope for good results. Time after time your cancer will beat you down.

Again and again you might end up with complications, infections, hospitalizations, and serious depression. It will take everything you have to keep yourself going in the right direction—towards the light. That is why at the end of my Journey, I have decided to compile some critical pieces of knowledge for you that will help you on your own Journey to beating cancer. Some of these are harsh realities, but I want you to know that they are important to consider.

Life changes perspective all the time. With cancer, you have good days and bad days. The trick is to fix the end goal of surviving in your mind and reach towards it with both hands. Listen to these pieces of advice, and add to them yourself. I strongly encourage you to record your Journey, as I did. With enough knowledge, perhaps one day a tome can be distributed to everyone in the world who gets cancer, and more people will survive and make it through that dark tunnel into the light. This is your time to educate yourself on what needs to happen. Whatever you need to do to survive through this time, you go ahead and do it. But remember that you are responsible for yourself. A few days of not eating can be disastrous with cancer. You *must* look after yourself like you are the King or Queen of the world.

Focus on Self Responsibility

- You have been diagnosed with cancer. It is the worst news you are ever likely to receive in your life. You know bad things are coming, but incredibly good things are also on their way. Never lose sight of the good things in your life. When I was diagnosed, the outpouring of love and support was heady. Focus on the good!

- Take responsibility for your body. You are going to need help, that is very true, but ultimately it is you who are responsible for your own survival. This is one of the very important things that I discovered on my long journey to being cancer free.

- No one knows your body better than you do. Everything you feel happens for a reason. *Never* ignore an ache, a pain, or something strange when you have cancer. If you do not know what it is, ask your doctor and get help. Do not allow other people to tell you it is something else, and do not believe what you read on the Internet. Find out from people who have actually medically trained for many, many years.

- Keep yourself clean to reduce your chances of getting infections. Shower every day, and wash your hands before and after every meal, outing, or bathroom break. Be as hygienic as you can be, and your body will thank you for it. This includes changing sheets, keeping your house clean, and brushing your teeth.

- Force yourself to eat three square meals a day that are packed with good nutrients. Stop eating junk food, and switch to vegetables and fruit with lean sources of protein. There will be days when you do not want to eat or drink, but you must do it. Do it despite yourself, and you will be strong enough to survive to the next trial.

- Focus on regaining strength where you can with exercise. Move while you can, even if it is only stretching. Get the blood flowing and the body going. I enjoyed walks, and it helped me survive. Find what you can do, and keep doing it until you cannot. You will spend time on your back. When you are not there, focus on exercise and strength.

Focus on a Support System

- No matter how positive you are now, days will come that tear you down. You must have a support system in place to help you survive: people who can drive you places, feed you, help you, and emotionally support you.

- Love is something I believe no cancer sufferer should be without. Find it where you can—with friends and family. I only had my friends around, but they showed me what real love looks like—caring, helping, and sharing the burden when someone really needs it.

- Happiness is essential because dark days are ahead. Serious times can cause depression quickly, especially when your health is involved. Fill your days with laughter, good spirits, and happiness, and deny stress. Feed your soul with happy things to make lightness out of heavy days; it makes all the difference.

- Reach out to the medical staff that is helping you. Get to know them, and do not be afraid to speak your mind. Share concerns, ask for information, and be resolute about staying informed every step of the way. My friends helped by taking notes, recording journal entries, and helping me make sense of the storm of information.

- Have people close to you that you can talk to about your day. Cancer is all consuming, so it will be the central focus until it is gone; there is nothing you can do but make up for that once you have won the fight. In the meantime, you need people around you to be strong, in good spirits, and willing to help you through tough emotions.

- Write things down if you find it helps you. This is also a great way to make sense of what is happening to you after it has happened. Share your experiences with support groups; find other cancer sufferers and connect. Chat to doctors, friends, and family—but do *not* suffer in silence. There is a time for being alone, and that time is *not* when you have cancer.

- Get support through books like this one. Read about other people's survival stories, and know that whatever the doctor has said, survival ultimately is up to you—no matter the statistic. You *can* survive, and survive you *must*.

Let Other People In

- There will be days when you need physical, mental, and emotional help. The following are some things you must do to make this easier on yourself.

- Let people pick up your slack at work, even if work is the center of your world. This is a battle for your life; you can always find a new job but not a new life.

- Let people cook and clean for you when you need it. They will see you at your best, and they will see you at your worst. They still love you, and they are there to help you, which means shutting up and accepting this help with love and respect.

- Let people motivate and inspire you. You will have days when you feel really bad and you do not know when it will end. This is when you need encouragement, motivation, and cheerful inspiration. Let your support wash over you, and take the reins of your happiness for a while until you are strong enough to care again.

- Depression will happen, along with anxiety. Neither of these things help you one little bit, but they creep in if you let them. Surround yourself with happy music, happy movies, and cheerful people and things. Horror or disturbing images can make depression and anxiety worse.

- Never underestimate the power of a friend coming to visit you. You will want to say no, but say yes! They remind you that life is still being lived and that you want to get back to that any way you can. Try not to turn away your friends and family.

- Smile, even if you do not feel happy. A mechanical smile automatically tells your body that you want to be more cheerful, and it works. Be grateful for the things and people that you have, and stop counting everything that is wrong with you. Instead, count the things that are right! Believe me, they outweigh the bad.

- Get involved in cancer awareness groups. It is all smoke and mirrors until it happens to you, but it really does matter that people are educated about it. Do not be afraid to tell people, because cancer will never define you. It is simply part of your life journey and an obstacle that you were always meant to overcome.

Some Final Pieces of Advice

- Sleep is vitally important when you have cancer, so make sure that you get enough of it. Lacking sleep will make you feel like death warmed up. If you cannot sleep, ask your doctor for help. This is no time to suffer in silence.

- If you disagree with your doctor, get a second opinion. If a medication does not work effectively or causes too many side effects, tell your doctor to change it! Doctors are there to help you, but they cannot do anything if you are keeping it to yourself. Speak up, speak loud, and stand up for the way that you feel.

- Tell your friends and family that you are officially a no-stress zone. Stress is a killer for cancer patients. It is stressful enough dealing with the disease; you do not need a whole pile of additional stress dropped at your feet. Keep it stress free.

- The Internet is brimming with bad, free information that has no merit. Most medical databases are locked behind permissions and payment gateways. Be careful what you trust, even if the site seems credible. By all means, ask your doctor, but do not be too quick to argue based on bad information that you got for free.

- It is a better course of action to seek out second and third opinions from other doctors in the same field than to use Dr. Google. In fact, Dr. Google can cause a lot more confusion and anxiety than you think. Leave it to the experts, but be strong enough to ask pertinent questions based on research and how you feel.

- Remind yourself that the end will come and that you will recover. It may be hard sometimes, but it is necessary. Cancer too shall pass. Time is on your side now; you just have to make it count by staying healthy and well fed and monitoring your every feeling.

- If in doubt, go to the hospital. You have cancer, and that is a good enough reason, even if you have stubbed your toe and it will not stop bleeding. Just go to the hospital and make sure that you are all right.

- Never stop fighting. Through your exhaustion, your depression, your pain—never give up on the light at the end of the tunnel. Track your progress, and be positive about what you have overcome at every step. Be your own biggest fan, and never surrender to cancer!

As a final note in my book, I want to extend the deepest and most sincere thanks I can afford to all of my friends and family who helped me get through my year with Stage 3 breast cancer. I beat it, and it was largely because of your faith, encouragement, prayers, and support every step of the way.

When you live day by day, the small things matter—a well-behaved son, a glass of water, a friend with a kind word. I will never be able to repay any of you for the light that you brought into my life during those tough times. With so much love and support, I am not surprised that I overcame this massive hurdle. I am now a cancer survivor, and you can be one too. Decide that you are going to live to tell others how you overcame this deadly disease, and give yourself the chance to make a difference.

We will all be impacted by cancer in one way or another; I really believe that. If we band together and spread awareness, we can help improve the lives of people all over the world who are currently living with this dreaded disease. Cancer will never define you, my friend, but it will make you stronger. It will remind you that life is for the living and that you have to fight to reclaim your place in the world that you built for yourself. Choose to *survive*.

Thanks again to my father, Frank, my mother, Henny, my brother, Franny, for the deep love and respect I have for you and how immensely proud I am to have you as my parents and my big brother! To my sons Gregory, Tye and Liam—I could not have asked for stronger children during this ordeal; you made Mama so very, very proud! You are my World, my Life, my Everything! You are my life's Work and Worth! To all of my childhood and longtime friends all across the U.S. and abroad, I thank you for following my Journey on the website faithfully and letting me know you had me in your thoughts and prayers. And to my local friends and all of my colleagues who became friends and family throughout this Journey—I am eternally grateful. I am nothing short of blessed to have you all in my life! To the doctors that worked tirelessly on making me well, even when my body had other ideas, I cannot express my gratitude enough. And finally, to you—the newly diagnosed cancer patient. Your journey is just beginning, but there is an end and a happy one at that. I hope my Journey has shed some light on what you can expect and has shown you that while you may go through a rollercoaster ride while on this cancer train, it does stop in the end. You can survive, and only you can determine how. Be your own greatest ally!

Never give up! Never surrender!

Gracie

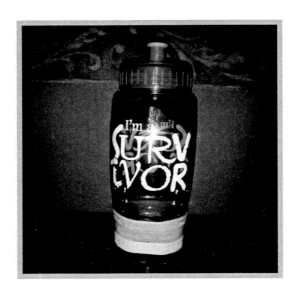

References

Positive Quotes, Brainyquote, http://www.brainyquote.com/quotes/topics/topic_positive.html

Chris Prestano, *Inspirational Quotes For Cancer Patients,* http://www.everydayhealth.com/cancer/inspirational-quotes-for-cancer-patients.aspx

Chris Prestano, *Inspirational Quotes For Cancer Patients,* http://www.everydayhealth.com/cancer/inspirational-quotes-for-cancer-patients.aspx

Quotations For Cancer Patients, Survivor and Loved Ones, Quote Garden, http://www.quotegarden.com/cancer.html

Quotations For Cancer Patients, Survivor and Loved Ones, Quote Garden, http://www.quotegarden.com/cancer.html

Quotations For Cancer Patients, Survivor and Loved Ones, Quote

Garden, http://www.quotegarden.com/cancer.html

nspirational Quotes, Brainyquote, http://www.brainyquote.com/quotes/topics/topic_inspirational.html

Inspirational Quotes, Brainyquote, http://www.brainyquote.com/quotes/topics/topic_inspirational.html

Inspirational Recovery Quotes, http://www.serenitypath.org/inspirationalquotes.html

Inspirational Recovery Quotes, http://www.serenitypath.org/inspirationalquotes.html

Inspirational Recovery Quotes, http://www.serenitypath.org/inspirationalquotes.html